MONTESSORI WORKS FOR DEMENTIA:

Everyday Activities For People Living With Dementia

Stephen Phillips and Bernadette Phillips BA MA Mont Dip Mont Cert

COPYRIGHT

Phillips, Stephen and Bernadette

MONTESSORI WORKS FOR DEMENTIA:
Everyday Activities for People Living With Dementia.

1. Montessori and Dementia 2. Activities for Dementia 3. Montessori
4. Montessori Activities 5. Montessori and Alzheimers

DISCLAIMER.
The activities in this book should be supervised. The authors of this book cannot accept any responsibility for any harm caused to any person in the carrying out of these or any related activities.

DEDICATION

To my nephew Alex Donnelly,
who inherited his mother's
"Heart of Gold".
Thanks for everything Alex.

AND

IN MEMORIUM

In memory of a beautiful lady named Verona, who at 85 did not
have dementia, but was a welcome visitor to my mother who does.

We will always remember the lovely times we shared with Verona,
drinking tea from the yellow tea-pot, and enjoying a slice or two
of cake, talking about our children and remembering times past.

It was a privilege to know Verona. We will remember her always.
May she rest in peace.

"The mental life of anyone who does not work at all is in grave peril."
Dr. Maria Montessori.

CONTENTS

Introduction.

INTRODUCTION

INTRODUCTION.

"The mental life of anyone who does not work at all is in grave peril."
Dr. Maria Montessori.

In May 1952, in Nordwijk in Holland, Dr. Maria Montessori, just three months short of her eighty second birthday was making plans, with her son Mario, to give yet another Montessori Teacher Training Course. Her biographer, Rita Kramer, writes: - "She had been thinking of making a trip to Africa, but it had been suggested that because of the state of her health she ought not to travel but arrange instead for her lectures to be given by someone else. Mario was with her and she turned to him and said, "Am I no longer of any use then?" An hour later she was dead of a cerebral haemorrhage." (Kramer p367). She had worked, quite literally up until the day she died.

Many of us will not be so fortunate to have the physical and mental capacities to continue working into our eighties. But, whether we are 40, 50, 60, 70, or even 80, Dr. Montessori's message was clear. The human being needs to have work, i.e. "meaningful activity" to carry out daily, because if he doesn't, he will very quickly atrophy and die.

The aim of this book is to show people what "meaningful activity" is, to explain why it is crucial for the mental health of the human being and to demonstrate how "meaningful activities" can be presented to people living with dementia, even in the later stages.

As this book is based on the discoveries of Dr. Maria Montessori, its purpose is to explain what the Montessori approach is and how that approach can help people living with dementia.

So let's get straight to it.

The Montessori approach refers to the body of discoveries made by Dr. Maria Montessori, who was a brain specialist, a surgeon, a general practitioner, a professor of the science of education and the full development of the human being, a pioneer in the area of special needs education, a founder of the Montessori method of education, a social activist campaigning for the rights of women and children, a world renowned humanitarian, a speaker at the Geneva Convention on education and peace, a recipient of the Legion of Honour, a three times nominee for the Nobel Peace Prize and an all round "good egg" and woman genius.

Dr. Montessori's discoveries about the human being are prolific and could fill libraries, let alone book shelves. For our purposes, we need to summarise the basic principles she discovered that apply to all human beings and then ask how can the application of these principles help people living with dementia.

People living with dementia have many problems, but they also have many strengths. These "strengths" are often buried and no one knows they are still there.

The Montessori approach can help people living with dementia by:

1) Finding out what their strengths and remaining abilities are.
2) Supporting those strengths and remaining abilities.
3) Building on those strengths and remaining abilities.

The Montessori approach is uniquely suited to doing this because of its emphasis on:

- Respect for the person as a unique human being.
- The prepared environment.
- Individual activity.
- Materials that are self-correcting.
- Progression from the simple to the more complex.
- Movement from concrete to abstract.
- Meaningful activities i.e "work".
- Independence.
- Opportunities for repetition of the task.

Layout of this book.
This book offers five categories of activities built around the five areas of human life that Dr. Montessori identified as being crucial to all humans. These activities are:

- Daily life Activities.
- Sensory Activities.
- Mathematical Activities.
- Language Activities.
- Cultural Activities.

Note:
The "procedures" in this book have been designed primarily for people who are living in the later stages of dementia. People with less severe dementia will find these tasks less challenging and may combine some of the steps in the "procedures" into one.

Also, many of the activities have 2 stages, a preliminary stage, where an indirect approach is used and a target stage where a direct approach is used.

An assessment of the person will dictate whether both stages are needed or whether the person would be able to go straight to the target activity.

Remember the Karate Kid, "wax on, wax off", well this is the same principle. Doing one activity such as scooping sweets from a bowl of lentils, is a very effective "indirect" way to get a person back into the habit of using a spoon to feed him/herself.

Similarly, pouring water from jug to jug is a very effective "indirect" way of getting a person back into the habit of doing many activities such as watering plants, pouring drinks into cups, pouring cream into coffee, pouring milk onto cereal, etc.

So, let's get started.

PART 1
UNDERSTANDING DEMENTIA

WHAT WE ALL NEED TO KNOW ABOUT DEMENTIA.

(Some Dementia Facts)

The World Alzheimer's Report 2014, states that:

"Dementia, including Alzheimer's disease, remains one of the biggest global public health challenges facing our generation. The number of people living with dementia worldwide today is estimated at 44 million."

However, that number is set to increase dramatically. In that same report, it states :

"By 2050, 135 million people around the world will live with dementia".

The financial cost facing society to provide care for this number of dependent people will be astronomical. The report further states:

"Given this epidemic scale, and with no known cure, it's crucial that we look at what we can do to reduce the risk or delay the onset of developing the disease.....as well as to promote the interventions to manage the quality of life of those living with it and their relatives."

The main purpose of this book is to promote interventions which hopefully will help to improve the quality of life for those living with dementia and their relatives.

With this in mind, our first task is to clarify to the ordinary man on the street, what dementia is, what causes it, how widespread it is, and what, if any, treatments are available for it. So, let's get straight to the facts.

What Is Dementia?

"Dementia" is an umbrella term used to describe symptoms that may include:

- memory loss
- confused thinking
- difficulty paying attention/concentrating
- difficulty with planning, organising and problem solving
- problems with language and communication
- disorientation
- visual perception problems

In addition to these problems which come under the heading of "cognitive symptoms," people living with dementia will often have problems associated with mood changes. They may become anxious, irritable, withdrawn, frustrated, easily upset or unnaturally sad and depressed.

Some people living with dementia may experience other symptoms as the illness progresses. These include: pacing up and down, asking repetitive questions and disturbed sleep. Physically, people living with dementia may experience weight loss as a result of lack of appetite and muscle weakness as a result of lack of movement, especially as they get older and are less mobile.

Are All Dementias The Same?

No, there are several different types of dementia. The most documented types are:

• Alzheimer's Disease:
This is the most common type of dementia. It accounts for about 50 to 80 % of dementia cases.

• Vascular Dementia:
This is the second most common type of dementia after Alzheimer's disease. It accounts for about 20% of dementia cases.

• Dementia with Lewy Bodies:
This is the third most common type of dementia after Alzheimer's disease and vascular dementia. It shares some of the symptoms of Alzheimer's disease and some of the symptoms of Parkinson's disease. It probably accounts for about 10% of all cases of dementia.

- Fronto-temporal Dementia.

This is one of the less common types of dementia, however it is a significant cause of early onset dementia i.e dementia in people between 45 and 65 years of age.

- Mixed Dementia:

The prevalence of this type of dementia is difficult to quantify as it can only be verified with certainty by autopsy. Mixed dementia refers to a situation in which a person has more than one type of dementia simultaneously. It is now believed by many experts in dementia that the prevalence of mixed dementia is probably significantly more common than was previously realised.

- Other Types of Dementia:

Any condition that causes damage to the brain or nerve cells can cause dementia. Some of these conditions are:

Parkinson's Disease
Huntington's Disease
Creutzfield-Jacob Disease

- Pseudo-Dementias or Reversible Dementias:

Certain physical illnesses mimic the symptoms of dementia, but when treated with the appropriate medications the symptoms of dementia lessen and sometimes disappear completely. Some of these conditions are:

vit B12 deficiency
hypothyroidism
adverse drug effects
alcohol abuse
normal pressure hydrocephalus

Certain mental illnesses, in particular certain types of depression, can mimic the symptoms of dementia. Persons with these conditions, may exhibit symptoms such as sleep disturbance, confusion, memory loss and other cognitive problems. However, when careful testing is carried out it is found that the person's memory and cognitive functioning are in fact intact. Persons diagnosed with these conditions often respond positively to antidepressants.

What Causes Dementia?

The causes of dementia vary according to the type of dementia. The main causes are as follows:

- Alzheimer's disease is thought to be caused by not one but a number of factors, which include age, genetic inheritance, environment, lifestyle, and overall general health.Although the causes of Alzheimer's disease are not yet fully understood, the damage it does to the brain is clear. Alzheimer's disease kills brain cells. The brain of a person with Alzheimer's disease has fewer cells and fewer connections among surviving cells than a healthy brain has. As more and more brain cells die, the brain of a person with Alzheimer's disease starts to shrink.The disease was named after Dr. Aloise Alzheimer, a German physician, who, in 1906, first identified the brain cell abnormalities that are now collectively referred to as Alzheimer's disease. While performing an autopsy on one of his former patients, who had died after years of suffering from confusion, severe memory problems and difficulties with language and comprehension, he noted particular brain abnormalities. These were; firstly, dense deposits surrounding the nerve cells (neuritic plaques) and secondly, inside the nerve cells, he observed twisted bands of fibers (neurofibrillary tangles). Even today, over 100 years since this discovery, Alzheimer's disease can only be physically diagnosed by autopsy.

- Vascular dementia is caused by problems with the blood supply to the brain. It may occur suddenly especially after a major stroke, or it may progress slowly over a period of time, usually after a number of "mini-strokes". A major stroke causes sudden restriction of blood flow to the brain resulting in brain cell death. Mini strokes cause tiny but cumulative damage. Over time, mini strokes or transient ischaemic attacks (TIAs) cause widespread damage to the brain.

- Dementia with Lewy bodies is caused by the build-up of tiny clumps, called Lewy bodies, which are protein deposits, inside brain cells. These clumps build up in areas of the brain which control muscle movement and memory. Why this occurs is still not fully understood.

- Fronto-Temporal Dementias are caused by the build-up of abnormal proteins in the part of the brain behind the forehead (the frontal area) and above and behind the ears (the temporal area). These abnormal proteins clump together and become toxic to the brain cells, causing them to die. Over time, the brain tissue in the affected lobes (frontal and temporal) shrinks. Why these abnormal proteins build up is not yet fully understood, but there is often a strong genetic link to their appearance.

• Other Types of Dementia are usually caused by specific medical conditions.

Who Gets Dementia?

Dementia mainly affects people over the age of 65. Some figures suggest that dementia affects one in 20 people over 65 and one in five people over the age of eighty. However, a significant number of people have early onset dementia, i.e. dementia which occurs long before the 65th year. Some dementias have a genetic cause and these types of dementia usually appear before age 65. Dementia affects both men and women. International research shows that dementia occurs in every country of the world. The World Alzheimer's Report, 2014, estimates that worldwide there are 44 million people living with dementia. This number is expected to increase to 135 million people by 2050.

How is Dementia Diagnosed?

Dementia is usually diagnosed by either a geriatrician, a neurologist or a psychiatrist. The diagnosis has to be based on a combination of factors because as yet, there is no single test for diagnosing dementia. These factors usually involve:

Firstly, taking a detailed medical history of the person's problems.
Secondly, cognitive testing, i.e. tests of the person's memory, his/her problem-solving skills, and general thinking patterns.
Thirdly, physical examination and tests to rule out other possible causes of the symptoms such as a specific vitamin or hormone deficiency.
Fourthly, a brain scan, this is usually how vascular dementia is diagnosed. The usual progression is for a person to be referred by their GP on to a specialist doctor or team who have expertise in dementia and so can carry out more specific tests and/or brain scans. The diagnosis is then explained to the person and their closest relative if possible.

How Is Dementia Treated?
As yet, there is no cure for dementia. All we can do is try to alleviate the symptoms. Treatments to alleviate the symptoms fall into two categories: drug treatments and non-drug treatments.

Drug Treatments.

There are a number of drug treatments which, especially if administered early on in the course of the disease, can not only help to ease the symptoms but also halt the progress of the disease for some time.

Some of these drugs may temporarily relieve memory loss and improve concentration and general interest in life for some persons with mild to moderate levels of dementia. Other drugs may be given to persons with later stage dementia to relieve symptoms of agitation, anxiety and delusion. People with vascular dementia will need to take drugs to control their blood pressure, cholesterol, heart or diabetic symptoms.

Non-Drug Treatments.

Many non-pharmacological therapies are used by care workers in the treatment of people living with dementia. These include:

- Aromatherapy and massage
- Music therapy and white noise
- Bright light therapy
- Psychological therapies.

Can We Prevent Dementia?

Since there is still a great deal of uncertainty about what actually causes dementia, it is difficult to know exactly how to prevent it.

However, since the causes of some dementias such as vascular dementia, are clear, there are steps we should take to try to avoid their development.

To help to prevent vascular dementia we should do what we can to help people to avoid strokes and mini-strokes. This involves controlling blood pressure, cholesterol, diabetes, and heart problems.

To help to prevent pseudo-dementias, we should help people to get early treatment for depression, vitamin and hormonal deficiencies.

To help to prevent Alzheimer's disease, we should encourage people to: eat a healthy diet, exercise, control weight, be socially active, exercise their brains through doing puzzles, crosswords etc. People should also be encouraged to avoid tobacco and excess alcohol.

WHY IS EVERYDAY LIKE GROUNDHOG DAY?

(Short-term Memory Problems In People Living With Dementia)

Several years ago I had my first visit to a "dementia" ward. A striking looking lady in her late 70s walked up to me, shook hands and introduced herself. She told me her name was Rebecca Wilcox, (not her real name) and that she was from "the Brontë country". She said her husband's name was Reginald P. Wilcox and her daughter Charlotte, her only child, was a university lecturer in London.

She chatted about her love of music, literature and art for about twenty minutes. Then she said she had to go off to have a rest. I was left thinking, what a lovely lady, but why on earth is she in here? She's so lucid and such an interesting person to talk to. She should be working here, not spending time as a resident!

About fifteen minutes later, I noticed at the end of the long corridor which led to the bedrooms, the same lady walking cheerfully in my direction. I smiled and waved and she waved back at me. She walked right up to me, shook hands, and introduced herself. She told me her name was Rebecca Wilcox and that she was from the Brontë country. She said her husband's name was Reginald P. Wilcox and her daughter Charlotte, her only child was a university lecturer in London.
I said, yes, I remember you telling me this a short time ago. She stared at me with a puzzled expression and said, "Were you here a short time ago? I don't remember meeting you, but it's nice to meet you now?"

I was there for a long time that day and I had a third encounter with this lovely lady which went pretty much the same as the first two. That was my first direct encounter with short term memory problems in people living with dementia.

This lady had so many "strengths". She could walk unaided. She had no mobility problems, indeed she had the stride of a ballet dancer. She could chat, joke and laugh at any amusing incident which took place. She could wash and dress herself unaided and braid her still beautiful white hair. She could choose from a menu what she wanted for breakfast, dinner and tea and she liked to read, do cross-word puzzles and listen to music. It appeared her only deficit was memory. She couldn't remember events that had just recently occurred.

Yet, to my shame, I now found myself focusing on her very obvious deficit. I was no longer thinking that she should be "employed" at the care-home instead of being a resident there. I started seeing only her problems. That, I now realise, is one of the biggest obstacles facing people who have been diagnosed with dementia. We start to focus on their deficits rather than their strengths. We, the onlookers, start to become anxious, nervous, terrified of what this condition could develop into. We start to see problems of all kinds ahead, and often, like a self-fulfilling prophecy, the problems start to appear. Yet the person living with dementia is often blissfully unaware that there is a problem, just like Rebecca Wilcox, who happily introduced herself to me three times, totally unaware that she was repeating herself, while I became tense and anxious.

I was like the Bill Murray character in the film Groundhog Day, who is exasperated by the insanity of having to live the same day over and over while the people around him are blissfully unaware that they are stuck in a time-loop.

This is a key problem in dementia, our unease. When we become agitated by the irrationality of it all, we send out signals that "all is not well," something is very wrong. In fact people living with dementia will often keep asking the persons caring for them "what's wrong?," "you're acting strange," "what's wrong?"

The person living with dementia is usually not aware that he/she is living in Groundhog Day, but we, the carers, are. And it is often we who unintentionally create a tense atmosphere. The person living with dementia is very sensitive to the atmosphere. Once they sense our tension, they become tense and a cycle of negative emotions arises, from which it is difficult for both the carer and the person living with dementia, to escape.

Now, we're not suggesting that anyone should be in denial about the very real problems facing people living with dementia, but we need to stop focusing on the problems as if that's all there is to the person. The person is "still in there", behind the problems.

So, what's the solution? Well, as yet, there is no cure for short term memory loss. So, until there is, perhaps we have to be like the Bill Murray character in the film, and put our time to good use while we are stuck for another day, another week, or another year, in "Groundhog Day".

WHY CAN'T MY MUM REMEMBER HOW TO MAKE A CUP OF TEA?

(Executive Function Problems In People Living With Dementia)

Someone very close to us is living with dementia. In fact, she is living with us while she's living with dementia. Let's call her Betty. Betty never drank alcohol, she never even tasted coffee and she only rarely drank fizzy drinks. But, she had a weakness for one drink......tea. Betty is an Irish person and Irish people love tea. The famous poet T. S. Eliot wrote about measuring out your life in coffee spoons. He wrote this to imply a note of sadness, a wasted life, but Betty, measured out her life in teaspoons and it wasn't sad or wasted. She loved her cups of tea and loved to put the kettle on the minute anyone came to visit her. She could have given "Mrs. Doyle", the housekeeper/tea-lady from the "Father Ted" comedy series, a run for her money!

Betty has vascular dementia, probably brought on by a series of mini strokes, which occurred over the years and could have gone undetected but for an MRI scan she had while in hospital getting treatment for a bout of pneumonia. Vascular dementia affects the front part of the brain, the part that controls what's known as "executive function". "Executive function," is a fancy name to describe the ability to perform important tasks such as: planning, making decisions, seeing consequences. But it also controls more down-to-earth things like remembering the sequence of steps for doing everyday tasks such as, putting your shoes on, getting dressed, and most importantly, making a cup of tea.

Now, hindsight is a great thing, but when life is actually happening, we don't have the benefit of hindsight. With hindsight, we now realise that some time ago, when Betty gave you a cup of tea and you found it was actually hot water with milk in it and no trace of a teabag, something was going wrong. And when Betty laughed and said "I must be losing my mind, imagine forgetting the teabag!" she actually was losing her mind. She was losing executive function which is part of the declarative memory system.

Memory is a fascinating phenomenon. We talk of "memory" as if it is just one mental ability, but memory is actually made up of a number of different types of mental abilities. Basically, we have two types of memory, short term memory, where we store memories of things which have recently occurred and long term memory where we store memories of things that have occurred in the past.

Long-term memory can be further divided into declarative memory i.e. ("knowing what") and procedural memory i.e. ("knowing how").

To put it simply, declarative memory is memory of facts or events that we consciously recall and bring to the forefront of our minds. For example, when we tell someone, "my name is X and my date of birth is XXXX and my telephone number is XXXX," we are using declarative memory. Specifically, in this example, because we are recalling information of a factual nature, we are using semantic memory which is a subcategory of declarative memory. If we said, "Hi, I'm Mary, remember we met at the grocery store last weekend," we would also be using declarative memory, but it would be another sub-category of declarative memory known as episodic memory, i.e. the type of memory which recalls specific things we have experienced, it is information of an autobiographical nature.

Another part of the declarative memory system is called "executive function." As we stated above, "executive function" is a term denoting the ability to plan, organise and make decisions. It also gives us the ability to understand the sequence of steps needed to perform many routine activities such as getting dressed in the mornings.

When a person is living with dementia, declarative memory is usually the part of memory that is most adversely affected. For this reason persons living with dementia may start to forget things of a factual nature like names, phone numbers, dates, even meanings of words, as their semantic memory becomes impaired. Similarly, persons living with dementia may begin to have difficulty recollecting specific events they have experienced as their episodic memory becomes impaired. And, if the executive function of a person living with the dementia is damaged, they may have trouble remembering the sequence of steps that are needed to carry out routine activities, and that probably explains why mum, "can't remember how to make a cup of tea."

NOTE

EVERY PERSON WITH MEMORY LOSS IS UNIQUE AND
WILL RESPOND DIFFERENTLY, AND EACH PERSON
CHANGES OVER THE COURSE OF THE CONDITION.

WHY CAN'T MY DAD REMEMBER THAT I VISITED HIM LAST SUNDAY?

(Episodic Memory Problems In People Living With Dementia)

Marsha's dad, Tom, is 79. He was diagnosed with Alzheimer's disease six years ago. One of the first signs that something was wrong was his gradual inability to remember events that had happened either recently or in the past. For example, over the past year when Marsha came to visit her dad and asked him "did you have lunch yet?", Tom couldn't remember. In fact he usually couldn't remember whether he had eaten breakfast either. He couldn't remember if he had taken his pills and he couldn't remember if he had received any phone calls from relatives.

Over the last year, he started to forget more significant events, such as Marsha's wedding which took place five years ago, the birth of Marsha's baby three years ago and the passing away of his own wife, Marsha's mother, one year ago. Tom also can't remember the fact that Marsha comes to visit him every Sunday.

These events, which Tom is unable to remember, are all part of his episodic memory and regrettably, episodic memory is often the first part of our memory system to become damaged by dementia.

What is Episodic Memory?
The term "episodic memory" was first coined by Dr. Endel Tulving in 1972. He defined episodic memory as "memory for personal experiences and their temporal relations.."
Episodic memory has to do with the, who, why, what, where and when of information storage. Examples of episodic memory include:

- Knowing who came to visit you in your home this morning.
- Knowing why you had to go to the A&E last week.
- Knowing what you had for lunch today in the cafe.
- Knowing when you first started to wear hearing aids.

Tulving proposed that episodic memory is a unique type of memory in that it involves "mental time travel" i.e. the feeling that we are going back in time in our mind's eye to revisit the scene of the event.

Not only that, but with episodic memories, we are consciously aware that we are recollecting something that is now past. We experience the "feeling" of remembering. Whether that recollection is a revisiting of the kitchen where we had a bowl of porridge this morning or the church we got married in five years ago or the hospital ward we spent time in last year, the recollection involves "mental time travel".

Episodic memory is also unique in our memory system in that it allows us to remember personal past events, entirely from our own perspective. For example, 50 people may attend a wedding and each of those 50 people will create an entirely personal episodic memory of that event.

One person may remember the smell of the fresh air and the apple blossoms on the walk up to the church door. Another may remember the sound of the church bells. Another may remember the shimmer of sunlight on the sequins of the bride's dress. Another may remember the tears in the eyes of the bride's mother. Another may remember the softness of the bride's skin as she kissed the guests after the wedding service. Episodic memory therefore is closely related to "autobiographical" memory.

Episodic memory also gives the human being the power of "episodic future thinking" i.e. the ability to mentally envisage the future. It makes possible "mental time travel" into the future as well as into the past. No other memory system has this same capacity. Tulving calls it, "a marvel of nature".

The fact that episodic memory involves not just the recollection of cold hard facts, but the personal, sensorial, recollection of an event, may provide us with an insight into how to try to retrieve these lost memories, even when a person is living with dementia and has suffered damage to his/her episodic memory.

Marcel Proust, the famous French novelist was the first person to coin the term "involuntary memory". This is the type of memory that "explodes" on us "out of the blue" when "cues" encountered in everyday life evoke recollections of the past without conscious effort.

In Proust's novel, A La Recherche du Temps Perdu, translated in English as, "In Search of Times Past," he describes how the taste of a little piece madeline cake dipped in tea inspired an "involuntary memory," which took him back years into the past, to his childhood when his aunt used to give him a madeline cake that she had first dipped into her own cup of tea.

He noted that the sight of the little madelines in the cake shop window had not brought back anything to his mind. It was the taste of the cake dipped in the tea that did it, having a powerful emotive effect on him making him feel intense happiness.

These "involuntary" recollections can be pleasant or unpleasant depending on what events they bring to the surface.

In my own experience, the sight and smell of a wide-brimmed cup of coffee takes me straight back to the street in Paris where I once spent a summer as an au-pair and floods my mind with the memory of the smells, tastes and sounds of the outdoor cafes in that specific street in Paris.

These memories usually trigger more "involuntary" memories, often bringing a flood of very specific episodes which I had long forgotten about, up to the surface.

Perhaps neurological research into "involuntary memory" holds a key to helping people living with dementia to retrieve episodic memories from their past.

However, until such breakthroughs occur, Marsha will just have to accept that it is damage to her father's episodic memory that continually prevents him from remembering that she visits him every Sunday.

NOTE

EVERY PERSON WITH MEMORY LOSS IS UNIQUE AND
WILL RESPOND DIFFERENTLY, AND EACH PERSON
CHANGES OVER THE COURSE OF THE CONDITION

WHY DOES GRANDMA KEEP FORGETTING MY NAME?

(Semantic Memory Problems In People Living With Dementia)

Josh is eight years old. He lives with his mum, his dad and his grandma. Josh has a very close relationship with his grandma. Since he was a baby, she played a big part in his life. She was the one who taught him how to ride a bike, how to splash in puddles, how to blow bubbles with his own saliva, how to get chewing gum off his shoes with ice cubes, and lots of other cool stuff. (Some stuff mum doesn't know about because she might get "grossed out".) Yes, Josh and grandma are as close as thieves. They go bug hunting together in the summer and they like to sip cocoa and marshmallows together, all cosy under the duvet in winter.

But, in the last two years something has changed in grandma. She can't seem to remember the names of things. She calls the remote control the "highery-lowery" thing. She calls Josh's bike his "wheely thing" and sometimes she can't remember Josh's name. She says it's "on the tip of my tongue" but she often can't remember it at all. But grandma is still a very cool granny and Josh just "fills in" the missing words for her.

So, what's going on with grandma? Well, last year she was diagnosed with Alzheimer's disease. She is in the very early stages and the only noticeable difference is her memory. What's happening is, the disease is affecting her semantic memory.

What is Semantic Memory?
Semantic memory refers to a part of long-term memory that acts as a database for the storage of memories of facts, concepts and names of objects, people and places that are not personal but are part of common knowledge. Semantic memory includes the memory of what the functions of things are. Examples of semantic memory would be:
- Knowing that snow is white.
- Knowing that London is the capital of England.
- Knowing that scissors are used for cutting things.

- Knowing that fridges are used for keeping things cold.
- Knowing that grass is green.
- Knowing that there are 12 months in a year.
- Knowing that kettles are for heating water.
- Knowing that Christmas falls on the 25th of December each year.
- Knowing that Josh's name is "Josh".

The concept of semantic memory was introduced in 1972 by Dr Endel Tulving. Dr. Tulving defined semantic memory as "a system for receiving, retaining, and transmitting information about the meaning of words, concepts, and the classification of concepts."

Semantic memory has been the subject of much research in recent years and the big question is: have the semantic memories been wiped out in the brains of people living with dementia or are they still there but the brain can't make the right connections to retrieve them?

The answer is not 100% clear yet. But one thing is clear. Most persons living with dementia have difficulties with semantic memory. They can no longer access facts and concepts that they had accumulated over their lifetime, either because they are wiped out or because they cannot be retrieved from their database. These facts involve everything from their knowledge of the capital cities of the world, their knowledge of the political parties of their country, their knowledge of the basic laws of their society, to the functions of ordinary, everyday objects, such as refrigerators, hairdryers, ovens, kettles, telephones, knives, forks and spoons.

The list is endless because it involves thousands of objects which their healthy brain had named and categorised over a lifetime. It also involves concepts such as what things are used for. Most importantly, it also involves remembering the names of your relatives.

The level of impairment in semantic memory differs from person to person living with dementia. For some people it presents very real problems and causes very real life changes. For others, it's just another annoyance and they just accept it and get on with life.

Grandma is one of those persons who just accepts it and gets on with life. So, until there is a cure for semantic memory problems, young Josh will just have to be on hand again to give his beloved grandma the "highery-lowery" thing when the TV channel needs changing.

NOTE

EVERY PERSON WITH MEMORY LOSS IS UNIQUE AND WILL RESPOND DIFFERENTLY, AND EACH PERSON CHANGES OVER THE COURSE OF THE CONDITION

HOW COME WE NEVER FORGET HOW TO RIDE A BICYCLE?

(Procedural Memory Strengths In People Living with Dementia)

We've been living in York, UK for a few years now. It's a beautiful city steeped in history going back to Roman times. One thing that stands out about York is the number of people riding bicycles. Bicycles are everywhere. Babies ride them, toddlers ride them, school children race along on them, and generally people from eight to eighty (and possibly beyond), cycle everywhere. Sometimes, when we've just waved to the third or fourth octogenarian cycling by, we find ourselves pondering the question - how come no matter how old we are, we never forget how to ride a bicycle? After all, we weren't born with the ability to cycle, it's not built in. Well, the answer lies in "muscle memory," or "procedural memory".

What is Procedural Memory?
Procedural memory, or "muscle memory," as it's sometimes called, is a type of long-term memory that involves the performance of actions that are so hardwired into the brain that they have become automatic. We've all heard the term "driving on automatic pilot," what is implied here is that an action is being carried out by someone who does not have to consciously think about the action, he just does it automatically.

Examples of actions carried out by the power of procedural memory would be:
• walking, without having to consciously think about it.
• talking, without having to consciously think about it.
• combing your hair, without having to consciously think about it.
• shaving without having to consciously think about it.
• riding a bicycle, without having to consciously think about it.
• driving a car, without having to consciously think about it.
• playing a musical instrument, without having to consciously think about it.
• singing a song, without having to consciously think about.
• reciting a poem, without having to consciously think about it.
• swimming a few strokes, without having to consciously think about it.

- typing on a keyboard, without having to consciously think about it.
- reading a book or magazine, without having to consciously think about it.

Now, the good news is, that because memory is located in various parts of the brain rather than in one part only, when dementia strikes, it doesn't immediately damage all of our memory systems. Neurology shows that the part of the brain which controls procedural memory is often "spared," that is, left undamaged in people living with dementia, despite the damage done to other parts of the brain which control other types of memory, such as episodic and semantic memory.

This is huge. This is where the potential for helping the person with dementia lies. If the person with dementia still has a fairly intact procedural memory then there is a window of opportunity available to us. Our job then, is to discover how we can use this remaining "strength" to allow the person living with dementia, to show us "who" they were and who they are now, especially if there is no relative there to tell us. We may be very surprised at what we discover.

This fascinating phenomenon has become a theme in films in recent years. A quiet unassuming man presents with amnesia. He doesn't remember his occupation or his name, yet he can sign his signature. Suddenly he is crossed by someone on the street and all of a sudden all hell breaks loose. The amnesiac floors the person, using trained assassin "moves" on him, suggesting that he is not "a quiet unassuming man" at all, but rather a secret agent of some kind. But how does he remember all those "defence moves" when he has amnesia?

The answer is they are stored in his procedural memory, his muscle memory, a part of the brain not affected by his amnesia. It's as if the memories are literally stored in his muscles or his very cells. That's really what procedural memory is all about. The memory has become part of our bodies, it is not just something stored in our heads. It is as if the memory has gotten into us at a cellular level.

Now most of the elderly persons we meet who are living with dementia will not have been "secret agents" in the past, but, in many ways they are "secret agents" now, in the present, because we don't know much about them and they may not be able to communicate with us. So, that's where procedural memory comes in.

It is through procedural memory that we will learn all about Dom and Henry and Betty and Cedric and Marie-Therese. Through procedural memory they will reveal to us "who" they really are. So, let's have a look at how the Montessori approach can "jog" the procedural memory and help people living with dementia to reveal to us who they were in the past and who they still are.

MONTESSORI-BASED PROGRAMMES FOR PEOPLE LIVING WITH DEMENTIA

"An aged man is but a paltry thing,
A tattered coat upon a stick, unless
Soul clap its hands and sing, and louder sing
For every tatter in its mortal dress."
W.B. Yeats.
Sailing to Byzantium.

The key word here is "unless".

In the early 1900s, Dr. Maria Montessori worked with mentally deficient children and she revealed to the world the heart-breaking conditions in which these human beings would be forced to live out their lives UNLESS there was a programme of carefully thought out interventions.

When she started to take mentally retarded children out of the asylums and through the painstaking application of her "brain science" taught them to hold a knife and fork, to dress themselves, to play, to write, to read, to pass the state exams, people of discernment could see that what Dr Montessori had discovered about the human brain was revolutionary. She had discovered that the human brain could be reorganised, reshaped, possibly even reconstructed, resulting in the transformation of people's lives.

Dr. Montessori went on to apply her "brain science" to the education of young children with normal brain function, older children, adolescents and university students. Had she lived longer, there is no doubt that she would have conducted experiments with the middle aged mind as well as the elderly mind. Sadly, she didn't get that chance.

History of Montessori Based Programmes For People Living With Dementia.

In the nineteen nineties, Dr. Cameron J. Camp, Director of the Centre for Applied Research in Dementia, Ohio USA, found that he was "beginning to see linkages between Montessori's approach and the translation of concepts in neuroscience into practical interventions for persons with dementia."

In 1999, he edited a book entitled "Montessori-Based Activities for Persons with Dementia" Volume 1.

This was a manual based on Dr. Camp's original idea of using Montessori-based programmes for people with dementia. The manual was made possible through the efforts of many individuals.

A second volume was published in 2006, again involving the talents of a large number of people who supported Dr.Camp's original idea.

Since then, certain gerontologists in the United States, Canada, Australia and parts of Europe have begun to use Montessori's ideas in their approach to the care of people living with dementia, both within care home settings and without, and the results are very encouraging.

Here then is a summary of what Montessori programmes for people living with dementia are all about.

The Term:
"Montessori - Based Programmes for People living with Dementia" is a term now used to describe an infinite number of individually planned programmes of activities which are designed to meet the needs of an individual or individuals living with dementia, through the use of the unique, "brain-based" approach known as the "Montessori Method."

The Aim:

The aim is to focus on the surviving "strengths" of the individual living with dementia rather than his deficits, and to create activities which will protect these "strengths" for as long as possible and even build on them.

The Approach:

The approach is exact and scientific. It involves:

- A very detailed assessment of the individual living with dementia, including details of his/her past likes, dislikes, interests and abilities.

- The creation of "a prepared environment."

- The creation of "tailor-made" activities which :

  - are heavily based on the procedural memory system, i.e. "muscle memory," rather than the declarative memory system, as procedural memory is the memory system most "spared" i.e. left undamaged, in dementia.

  - make use of established rehabilitation principles and techniques such as:
    - Task breakdown.
    - Repetition.
    - Progression from the simple to the complex.
    - Progression from the concrete to the abstract.

- The use of few or no words in the presentation of the activity. Verbal instructions, if they are needed should be short, simple and pleasant.

- The use of a much reduced "tempo" in the presentation of activities. We need to learn to slow down to the pace which suits the person living with dementia rather than the pace which most suits ourselves.

- The use of materials which:

  - are self correcting. i.e. have a built in control of error.

- isolate the area of difficulty, i.e. if the activity is about matching colours, the pieces of the activity should be identical in every respect except colour, so they draw the person's attention to the "area of difficulty," i.e. "colour."

- The use of positive reinforcement if looked for, i.e, if the person looks for confirmation that he/she is doing the activity correctly, positive feedback and encouragement should be given to enhance the person's feelings of self-esteem because it is the process that is important not the end result.

- The use of repetition of an activity to promote positive engagement and the possibility of new learning.

- The use of indirect activities as a means of "priming the pump" of procedural memory in order to help the person to move towards carrying out the "target skill," e.g. getting the person to use dressing frames in order to "prime the pump" of muscle memory so that he/she will start dressing himself/herself again.

- The use of materials that do not offend the dignity of the person, i.e are not childish.

- The use of a no-correction approach. The purpose of the activities is to help the person to retain and possibly strengthen their remaining skills, it does not matter very much if the person makes mistakes. The emphasis should be on encouraging the person to do things for themselves again. Correction, of any sort could discourage the person and dissuade them from even trying any activities.

The Principles:

Montessori-Based Programmes for people living with dementia are based on a number of key principles that form the essence of Dr Montessori's discoveries about the human being. These principles are:

KEY MONTESSORI PRINCIPLES

"Independence"

The human being cannot feel fully human unless he/she is independent, i.e. able to do things for himself. Independence is a law of life.

"Work"

The human being cannot feel fully human unless he/she has opportunities to do work i.e. meaningful activities. Work is a law of life.

"Respect for human dignity"

The human being cannot feel fully human unless he/she is treated with respect, and his dignity as a human being, is recognised. Respect for one's dignity is a vital human need.

"Self esteem"

The human being cannot feel fully human unless he/she has a sense of self esteem. Self esteem cannot be purchased, or given as a gift. The human being attains self esteem by accomplishing tasks.
Self esteem is a vital human need.

"Contribution"

The human being cannot feel fully human unless he/she is given opportunities to contribute to the world he finds himself in. Contribution to the world we live in is a vital human need.

"Intergenerational Living"

The human being needs to live in the midst of a wide variety of age groups. This is a vital human need.

Many people are not aware of Dr. Montessori's views on the need for intergenerational living. Montessori wrote: "Nothing is duller than a Home for the Aged. To segregate by age is one of the cruellest and most inhuman things one can do." "The charm of social life is the number of different types that one meets."

(The Absorbent Mind p226).

Examples of Montessori Activities For People Living With Dementia.

• Using dressing frames to stimulate the "muscle" memory of fastening buttons, zips and buckles so as to aid persons with dementia to dress themselves again thereby giving the persons a sense of independence and self-esteem.

• Scooping small objects hidden in a bowl of rice with a sieve spoon, in order to stimulate the "muscle" memory of spooning so as to aid persons with dementia to feed themselves again thereby restoring dignity to those persons.

• Pouring liquids from one jug to another in order to stimulate the "muscle" memory of pouring so as to aid persons with dementia to carry out real tasks such as serving drinks to others, thereby helping the persons to feel a sense of usefulness in the community.

• Using a light hammer and a peg board with wooden pegs to stimulate the memory of hammering in a person who used to do handiwork so as to evoke memories from the past and also to enable the person to carry out light handiwork again thereby helping the person to feel useful once more.

• Using play-dough and cookie cutters to stimulate the memory of rolling out pastry so as to aid the person to start baking again and thereby feel a sense of being useful and of contributing to community or family life.

The Evaluations:
Statistical evaluations have been collated over the past few years and all of them are positive showing higher levels of engagement and happiness in persons who are participating in Montessori Based Programmes for people living with Dementia. However, instead of listing statistics, let's look at some real people.

• **Shirley:**
In one centre for people living with dementia we read about Shirley, aged 73, a former school teacher, who is offered the job of grading the maths work of 5 and 6 year olds from a local Montessori school. This "job" addresses the cognitive part of the Montessori for dementia programme at the centre. The therapist working with Shirley says: "There is a misconception that patients who have been diagnosed with dementia can no longer learn or be productive....That's simply not true. This approach helps stimulate their minds while also helping them maintain their current abilities."

This particular job was designed specifically for Shirley to evoke memories and experiences from her past.

• Harry:

Harry, a former GP, spends hours writing out "prescriptions" on a note-pad, thereby evoking pleasant memories of a career he pursued for a life-time. Out of this activity, he derives a feeling of self-worth and usefulness.

• Matt:

Matt, a former plumber works with plastic piping, thereby bringing back memories of the trade he pursued for a lifetime, helping him to feel useful and productive.

• Lucy:

Lucy, a former waitress, spends hours setting tables with placemats, small vases of flowers and serviettes which she folds herself.

All of these activities are planned out and "prepared" earlier by Montessori trained carers who make sure that each activity is offered in carefully prepared stages. There is a progression from simple to complex in the activities and there is minimum chance of failure built into these activities. For example, Lucy's placemats have been carefully designed with a silhouette of a knife, fork, spoon and plate on them so that they act as a template for Lucy as she lays out cutlery and plates on the table.

Activities are a mixture of the practical, sensorial, mathematical literary and cultural. Cultural activities especially those involving music have been shown to have great success in "awakening" a person living with dementia from states of apathy and inactivity to states of liveliness, smiles, laughter, song and even dance. Let's look at some real people.

• Dom: (Rediscovering your "joy," through the power of music).

In their beautiful book, "You say Goodbye and We say Hello," Tom and Karen Brenner, two experts in dementia, give a vivid example of procedural memory in action.

They tell the story of Dom, a person living with dementia in a locked dementia unit in a care home. They explain that "Dom had been a pianist and a choral teacher all of his adult life." When they met him he had "become withdrawn, belligerent and difficult to deal with". But, they witnessed first-hand how "when he sat down at the piano in the gathering room of the long term care home, he could play tunes from memory for hours!" Tom and Karen describe how;-

"He was a wonderful musician who played with flourishes, panache and with great joy. His whole face would light up and he would become lost in the music. People would spontaneously gather around the piano and join in the singing as Dom played." Tom and Karen write;-

" Dom was a happy man when he sat down to play the piano. That was the only time we ever saw him being gregarious, relaxed and happy. Music was the one thing that seemed to reach him. Through the music Dom gave himself and many others hours of unadulterated joy." p134

Tom and Karen then go on to talk about drum circles and how they use them to connect with people living with dementia. Tom and Karen's book is a must read for anyone interested in understanding dementia and how "we can" reach into the souls of the human beings trapped inside this cruel illness through their procedural memory which is still intact enough to be able to respond to the rhythms of music.

• **Henry: (Becoming animated again, through the power of music).**

Recently, a clip on the internet "went viral" showing the astonishing effects of music on an elderly man named "Henry" in a nursing home. Henry rarely spoke and often looked apathetic and lethargic just sitting in his chair. Yet when a care worker put a set of headphones on him and played his favourite music on an iPod, he started to sing along and move to the music. He became revitalised and communicative. He gave coherent and lively answers to the carer's questions. He talked about his favourite music. Neurologist Dr Oliver Sacks, commenting on the video said: "In some sense Henry is restored to himself. He has remembered who he is and has re-acquired his identity for a while through the power of music."

• **Betty: ("Staying Alive," through the power of music).**

I'm sitting at home watching an old Bee Gees concert on DVD with my 84 year old mother who is living with dementia. The brothers are singing songs from the films "Saturday Night Fever" and "Grease" and in the background they are showing clips from the films on a giant screen. My mother, who had been showing no interest in anything today, is suddenly very animated. She is starting to move to the music and has begun to tap her hands on her knees to the rhythm of "Grease is the word, is the time, is the moment, grease is the way we are feeling."

She is smiling and laughing at the video clips and clapping along at some of the disco-dance songs. We end up watching the entire concert twice! At the end of the second showing, and after about twenty cups of tea, she comments, "I hope they show that again tomorrow, the singing is really lovely, it's just one good song after another." Then she says, "it makes you feel alive."

I find myself unable to reply. All I can think of is why do we spend so much of our time writing about all the negatives in dementia, instead of snatching the positives and working with them and milking them for all they are worth? Why are we so limited in our vision? Well, I know the answer. It's because we get so tired and weary just dealing, day after day, with the realities of the negatives. But let's take heart. Let's see what we can do with "the power of music in dementia."

• **Marie-Therese: (Remembering your heritage through the power of music).**

A few years ago, I was asked by a young carer in a nursing home to come up to a locked unit to see a lady with severe dementia. The lady was originally French although she had lived in England for many years. The dementia had robbed her of language, and although she had been in the care home for several years, no one had ever heard her speak any language. She just grunted or screamed. The care worker had heard somewhere that I spoke French and hence my invitation.

I came along as asked, but before entering the lady's room, the care worker warned me to be very careful. She warned me that the lady who was bed ridden and had to be hoisted to be washed was usually very aggressive and if she grabbed hold of my hand, would probably bite me, with her few remaining sharp teeth.

I was a little nervous, but entered the room. I didn't speak or even look directly at the lady, I just started to hum the lyrics of a French mediaeval song that I had learned in my teens. It had a very soft, rhythmical sound to it and very repetitive words. I just kept singing it very quietly. The young care worker with me looked dumbfounded but thankfully she said nothing, she just stood silently beside me. Within a few minutes, the lady, who had started screaming when we entered the room, quietened down to a complete silence. All you could now hear in the room was the sound of my voice repeating the chorus of French words over and over. I was almost in a trance. I didn't know where the words were coming from. I was not even consciously aware that I still remembered this song from over 30 years ago, but I just kept on singing. The lady was staring at me now. Something had obviously been triggered in her brain. It was as if she'd had an electric shock.

She focused on me like a hawk on a mouse. I looked at her directly now and moved closer to her. I could see that she must have been a very beautiful woman in her youth, she still had high cheekbones and piercing green eyes. She started to move her mouth into a kind of smile, revealing a few very even front teeth. I just kept singing. My companion, the young care worker, stood still as if at a performance, and then slowly, as if in slow motion, began the work of washing and dressing the lady. I joined in the work, still softly singing. When the lady was washed and dressed, myself and the care worker left the room. Neither of us spoke. Before I left the room, I had whispered "au revoir" to the lady, and a quick "a demain", (until tomorrow).

Later that day, the care worker, came to me to tell me that she had never seen the lady like this before. The singing had somehow touched something inside of her and calmed her. The carer said: "she's peaceful as a sleeping baby even now, even though its hours since your visit". The care worker asked me if I would come back to see the lady another day. I said I would.

A few days later, as it was nearing Christmas time, the carers in that home had prepared a room with a very large Christmas tree, and a fireplace with Christmas stockings hanging on it, and were bringing the residents, in small groups down to this cosy room to sing carols and have mince pies and tea. I was asked to come to one of these gatherings in the hope of being able to give some company to this French lady.

Only one resident had turned up so far, so it looked like it was going to be a quiet gathering. I was sitting on the floor beside the fireplace wrapping small presents for the residents when Marie-Therese was wheeled into the room in her wheelchair.

As she came in, I just knew she had spotted me out of the corner of her eye. I was right, she did an about turn and looked straight at me. I know she recognised me. I continued to sit on the floor and wrap the presents, humming the same French medieval song that I had sung a few days earlier. Marie Therese stared at me. Slowly I got up and very cautiously moved nearer to Marie Therese and sat in the chair beside her. I passed her a drink and a small piece of mince pie.

She sipped the drink and I started to talk to her about Christmas. I wished her a "joyeux noel". It was a one-sided conversation for about 20 minutes. Then something remarkable happened. Marie-Therese spoke! She had never spoken before and everybody thought she couldn't speak. I didn't understand what she said to me but I knew it was French, so I replied in French. I kept talking about ordinary things, my name, where I came from, how I love Christmas, how I love snow, etc. She listened and then spoke again. I will never forget what she said. It was, "C'est horrible ce cafe." - "This coffee is horrible." Well, I did say she was French, and only the French know how to make good coffee!

So, we had a real breakthrough. I had one more visit with Marie Therese, after Christmas, and this time, I thought I'd go for a song she must know,- The Marseillaise, the French national anthem. I'll never forget the look on the carer's face when I broke into- "Allons enfants de la patrie, le jour de gloire est arrive..." completely out of the blue, but what I most remember is the sight of Maria-Therese's lips moving as she mouthed the words with me. I was too choked up to sing it to the end.

Unfortunately, I was unable to keep up my contact with Marie-Therese, but I will never forget her. She taught me a priceless lesson and that is: deep within our subconscious, in the area of procedural memory, we have stored vast amounts of treasures. These may be snippets of tunes we heard when we were kids, snippets of songs we sang when we were lovesick teenagers, snippets of lullabies we hummed as we paced the floor with a sleepless infant, and even snippets of our National Anthems which we learned with pride when we were young.

What Marie-Therese taught me is that these treasures are most likely not lost. They are locked in the recesses of the brain just waiting for someone to find the key or keys to release them. The power of song may well be one of the keys that does just that.

• **An un-named Lady: (Becoming a person again, - by the power of reading).**

In his wonderful book, Hiding the Stranger in the Mirror, Dr. Cameron Camp tells a very interesting story about reading and people with dementia. He tells how he was at an assisted living community for persons with dementia. He was about to provide some training to hands-on care staff when a resident with advanced dementia came into the room the staff were entering. The resident wore an apron with pockets, all stuffed with "collectables" she had gathered in her wanderings around the facility - eating utensils, knick-knacks, etc. He says the woman was completely silent as she walked up to a table and sat down in a chair next to a staff member. He says nobody paid any attention to the lady until he handed her a book about Gene Kelly, opened it to the first page, and said, "What does this say?" The woman proceeded to read the entire page out loud. He says he could not help but notice that the staff member sitting next to the lady appeared startled. He thanked the resident for helping read the story, and she then smiled and left the meeting. He asked the staff member nearby why she was startled when the resident read the page. The staff member said, "I didn't even know that she could talk."

Dr. Camp writes: "The point of these examples is that reading is a habit. We just do it, often without thinking about it. It is a habit, it is an ability that is seen in many persons with dementia, even in its advanced stages." p35

When people are elderly and they are living with dementia, we tend to become so focused on the things they can't do that we forget all about the things they can do. One of these things is the ability to read. People living with dementia should be given opportunities to read either on their own or with someone who could perhaps chat about the book or the magazine they are reading. It is remarkable that the ability to read is a strength that often remains intact even in persons living with advanced dementia. Reading a passage often leads to a follow-up conversation allowing the person living with dementia to communicate his/her feelings, memories or opinions. As such it is vital that we milk this remaining strength for all it's worth.

• **Cedric: (Re-living your history through the power of words).**

Cedric was in his eighties. He had late stage dementia and lived in a care home. He couldn't speak, as far as any one knew, and for the past few months, seemed to be really slipping way into an abyss of silence and immobility.

One afternoon, as he lay half asleep in an armchair in the communal room, a lively resident suddenly shouted out:

> "we shall fight on the beaches,
> we shall fight on the landing grounds,
> we shall fight in the fields and in the streets,
> we shall fight in the hills;
> we shall never surrender....".

Before he got any further, Cedric had bolted up and was standing strong shouting:

> "we shall fight on the beaches,
> we shall fight on the landing grounds,
> we shall fight in the fields and in the streets,
> we shall fight in the hills,
> we shall never surrender....."

The only other staff member in the room besides me, was a young care-worker who I think was too young to appreciate the significance of these words. But even she was rendered speechless.

The incident was remarkable but it was over as quickly as it began. Cedric sat back down and went back to sleep in the armchair.

The words were from one of Winston Churchill's famous speeches to the nation of Great Britain during the second world war and they hold huge importance and emotional significance for any British person and rightly so.

No one in the care home knew whether Cedric had played an active role in the war. He may well have. Many British men of his age did. These words certainly meant something to him.

Sadly, Cedric passed away a few days after this incident.

Perhaps if someone had known a little more about him they could have read some of Winston Churchill's speeches to him and perhaps he would have joined in as he did on that day when he made that remarkable impromptu speech.

So, what we see in all of this is that an aged man could be "just a paltry thing", a "tattered coat upon a stick", UNLESS we help his soul to sing and "louder sing for every tatter in its mortal dress".

At this point in time, Montessori Based Programmes for people living with Dementia are being designed to do exactly this and we believe they point the way forward towards how we might successfully "help the human being in the later years".

Epilogue:

Maria Montessori started her life's work in the area of brain dysfunction. It was pathology she was working with, not health. Through her dogged persistence and painstaking hard work she managed to break through into the chaotic mind of the mentally retarded child. She broke through the walls of silence, the screaming, the crying, the erratic behaviours, the biting, the aggression, the grabbing onto others, the pacing up and down, the hand flapping, the head-banging, the constant attempts to "escape."

Through her genius she was able to transform the quality of the lives of thousands of so called "idiot" children. Most of these children were never completely "cured" but their lives were enhanced, given meaning, given purpose, and they were afforded an opportunity to make their contribution, in whatever way they could, to the world they found themselves in.

We believe that Montessori-based programming for people living with dementia has the potential to do exactly this. It may never "cure" dementia, but it has the potential to enhance, to give meaning, purpose and a sense of human dignity to the millions of people who are living with dementia. It has the power to uncover the human being behind the illness, even though for some, this may only be for a few fleeting moments in time.

Since this work builds on the genius of the woman named Maria Montessori, we think it is fitting to conclude this section with her words:

"I set to work feeling like a peasant woman who, having set aside a good store of seed-corn, has found a fertile field in which she may freely sow it. But I was wrong. I had hardly turned over the clods of my field, when I found gold instead of wheat; the clods, concealed a precious treasure. I was not the peasant I thought myself. Rather I was like Aladdin, who, without knowing it, had in his hand a key that would open hidden treasures."

(The Secret of Childhood) p121

We, the joint authors of this book, believe passionately, that Montessori based programming for people living with dementia is a "key" that can open "hidden treasures" in our ongoing battle to find solutions for the millions of people throughout this world who are living every day of their lives, with dementia.

PART 2
EVERYDAY LIFE ACTIVITIES

CARE OF ONE'S SELF

- Washing

- Dressing

- Grooming

- Eating

- Toileting

CARE OF ONE'S SELF.

Things To Ponder.

Dementia is a disability that can go undetected for a long time. Even the person who actually has it, may not know it. However, one area that often gives a clue to family and friends that their loved one has dementia is when the person stops taking personal care of themselves.

Taking care of yourself involves many things. In this book, we are addressing specific areas of personal care such as washing, dressing, grooming, eating and toileting.

These are what you might call "private" areas of personal care. Most people don't involve others in their daily washing, dressing, or grooming habits, and they certainly don't involve others in their toileting routines.

Now, when someone develops dementia, and begins to have very real difficulty carrying out these daily routines, they often try one specific approach and that approach is called the - "cover it up and it might go away" approach.

The "Cover it Up" approach.
The person living with dementia can feel so demoralised because they now recognise that they have very real difficulty washing, dressing, grooming, going to the toilet, and sometimes even feeding themselves, that they do the first thing that occurs to them, i.e., "cover it up". They do this for a number of very valid and very intelligent reasons which often include:

1) Fear.
The person living with these problems is fearful that if family or friends find out the extent of their problems they may put them in a nursing home, causing them to have to leave everything that is familiar to them, everything that has been their life and their home, often for more than 50 years. None of us can really grasp the awful significance of this. Since, this would be a hugely daunting prospect for most of us with our full faculties, we can only just imagine what it must be like for someone who is experiencing mental confusion at the same time.

2) Embarrassment.

The person living with these problems often feels huge embarrassment around the whole area of washing, dressing, grooming and especially toileting. The person is aware that he/she is now experiencing real practical difficulties carrying out these tasks and because the person is so embarrassed about anyone finding out about the extent of these difficulties, the person decides on what he/she sees as a safe course of action and that is - "don't do them". He/she makes a clear decision: "don't wash, don't dress, don't groom, then you won't subject yourself to the frustrations of not being able to do these tasks properly and you'll save yourself from the embarrassment of being exposed as someone who's not capable anymore of doing even these most basic of life skills.

There are probably many more reasons why people living with dementia try to "cover up" their limitations, but these are the chief ones.

Our job then is to help the person to re-learn how to do these daily tasks again and so eliminate their fears and sense of embarrassment and demoralisation.

The Good News

The good news is that there are ways of helping people to re-learn how to perform their own personal care once again, even if they need some help with it. And the best news is, that when people start to do these things for themselves again, e..g. washing, dressing, grooming, they re-build their self-esteem which has no doubt taken a battering because of the onset of this cruel illness.

All of us feel better after we've had a shower or a wash, combed our hair, brushed our teeth, and the older person, living with dementia is no different.

We must help these persons to feel once again the pleasure of feeling clean and fresh, well groomed and tidied up.

Much of what we need to do involves preparation, meticulous planning and patience, patience, patience.

So, let's get started.

WASHING

Things To Ponder.

Most persons living with dementia have been washing themselves independently for over fifty years. But now, as a result of this disability they face a host of problems associated with the activity of washing. Some of these problems are:

- A lack of motivation to wash themselves.

- An inability to "call up to memory" the steps involved in washing.

- A sense of anxiety about the whole process of washing.

- An irrational fear of washing - ablutophobia.

- A physical inability to wash themselves.

Let's take a detailed look at each of these problems.

1) Lack of motivation.

One of the major problems encountered by people living with dementia is that the illness can rob them of motivation, even the motivation to get up and wash themselves. This is not a choice he/she makes. The illness is the root cause of this lack of motivation. Family members are often shocked by the person with dementia's lack of interest in washing themselves, or even worse, their flat refusal to wash. The matter can quickly become more of a problem for the family members or carers than for the person with dementia. The reasons for this are obvious. The family member or carer does not want to appear to be neglecting the care needs of the person with dementia. However, the person with dementia, can't really comprehend why his/her not washing is anyone else's business and usually considers that it is an outrageous invasion of his/her privacy that anyone other than him/herself should even address the issue.

2) An inability to remember the sequence of steps involved in washing.
This is something that is not widely known even by family members looking after a person with dementia, but it is a crucial fact affecting every aspect of the person with dementia's daily needs. The fact is this: the person living with dementia often cannot "call up to memory" the procedures or steps needed to have a wash or a shower. This is because the illness often damages the frontal cortex part of the brain, that is the part of the brain responsible for "executive function" i.e. decision making and also, most importantly, for helping the person to remember the sequence of steps needed to carry out everyday activities. Confusion over the steps, coupled with anxiety, which is a hallmark of many types of dementia may cause the whole issue of washing to become a fraught one.

3) A sense of fear and anxiety about the whole process of washing.
This is something that the person without dementia finds very difficult to understand. Why should washing yourself be such a fearful activity? What's all the palaver about? Why is the person creating such a fuss about nothing? These are all the exclamations we make when we are faced with trying to get a person with dementia who refuses to wash into a bathroom. But, you know what, the fuss isn't about nothing. A person with dementia can have a very real sense of fear and anxiety about the whole process of washing for the following reasons:

a) memory problems: the person is often fearful of taking off their clothes in case they can't remember where they put them and so may never find them again.
b) privacy issues: the person often fears that their privacy and dignity will not be respected and that they may have to strip off in the view of others.
c) sexual abuse: many elderly people were abused in childhood and because abuse was tolerated and often kept secret by both children and adults alike, the harm caused was never brought to the surface and so never dealt with. In circumstances such as this, it is natural that an elderly person with dementia would feel very vulnerable in relation to the whole idea of undressing to wash.

4) An irrational fear of washing - ablutophobia.
This is an uncommon but serious phobia, involving an irrational fear of bathing, washing or cleaning. The person feels total panic at the very prospect of bathing.

5) A physical inability to wash themselves.
As dementia progresses through its various stages, the person living with it can gradually lose the physical ability to do things. The person living with dementia is caught up in a vicious cycle. The illness robs him/her of the motivation to do physical activity. Lack of activity causes the muscles to waste. So a person in late stage dementia may not have the physical ability to wash him/herself.

The Good News.

None of these problems are insurmountable. Using a combination of common sense and Montessori Principles, we may be able to come up with solutions to the problems of:

1) How to deal with the "lack of motivation".

2) How to deal with the "inability to remember the steps involved in washing".

3) How to deal with the "sense of anxiety about the whole process of washing".

4) How to handle ablutophobia.

5) How to handle the physical inability to wash.

So, let's get started.

4)   How to deal with the problem of "lack of motivation".
Let's take a look at how Dr. Montessori managed to inspire "street" children who were not initially motivated to wash themselves, to develop an interest, one might even say a "joy" in washing themselves.

Dr. Montessori found that a major key to her success in this area lay in the materials she used, so let's examine this aspect of care.

The Materials we use.
Dr. Montessori found that when the materials used were simple, uncluttered, and painted in attractive but not overpowering colours, they attracted the attention of the children. It was as if they called out to the children subliminally, whispering thoughts in their heads like, "use me", "handle me", "try me".

Dr. Montessori paid particular attention to the physical size of the children and the materials used. She ordered little bars of soap that fitted perfectly into the little children's hands. She had little wash stands made to suit the heights of the children. She bought small attractive towels for the children to dry their hands in which hung on attractive low hooks easily accessible to the children because of their strategically low position. Everything about her little wash stands sent out subliminal messages to the children saying - "use me", "try me out", "wash with me".

Now, with regard to people living with dementia, we need to do exactly the same. We want the "washing materials" to send out an unconscious signal to the person which says - "wash with me". This will not happen if we offer the person a wash in a clinical looking white plastic basin or if we lead them kicking and screaming to a shower in a wet room that looks cold and uninviting.

It is well worth remembering that a person in their 80s who is living with dementia would have been born in the 1930s and therefore would, most likely, have grown up in a home without electric showers or even baths. In the 30s, 40s and 50s many homes did not even have an indoor toilet or bathroom The toilet was often located outdoors in a type of shed and the bath was a portable unit that was kept behind a curtain in a scullery in the kitchen.

Now, a person in their 80s may have had an electric shower in their home for the past 40 years, but if they are now living with dementia and the illness causes them to think they are living in the days of their childhood, they will not find electric showers very familiar at all and may, in fact, be very frightened of them.

For this reason, it may well be more appropriate to make a little portable "washstand" for the person with dementia. This stand would have three simple items placed on it: a pewter jug of warm water, a ceramic bowl to pour the water into and a little bar of soap on a ceramic soap dish.

The sight of the jug and ceramic bowl may or may not bring back memories to the person with dementia, but the physical act of pouring water from the jug to the bowl may "jog" the person's procedural or "muscle memory" causing them to "call up to memory" the recollection of the physical movements associated with pouring water into a bowl to have a wash.

The use of "old fashioned" materials like a pewter jug and ceramic bowl may also involve the person's "involuntary memory", flooding him/her with recollections from the past, just like what happened to the person in Marcel Proust's novel referred on pages 14 and 15.

Remember, it was not the sight of the little madeline cakes that brought back the memories to the person, but the process of dipping the piece of madeline cake in the tea and then tasting it. Similarly, the person with dementia may show no sign of remembrance at the "sight" of a washstand with a ceramic bowl and pewter jug. Moreover, the person may not "semantically" remember what washing means, but, observing someone washing with these materials or even trying them out him/herself may "jog" the person's "muscle memory" and their "involuntary memory" together, thus calling up to their mind the recollection of holding a pitcher of warm water and pouring it carefully into a ceramic bowl in order to wash. They may "call up to memory" the long forgotten sensation of rubbing the bar of soap between their hands. They may "call up to memory" the long forgotten smell of the bar of Pears or carbolic soap. All of these recollections are not evoked through "semantic memory", but through procedural or "muscle memory" aided by the "involuntary memory".

So, what we are looking at here is a new way of helping the person to "remember" by the use of specific and carefully prepared materials. We are not trying to evoke recollections from the person's semantic or episodic memories because these are the parts of memory that are most damaged by dementia. Instead, we are trying to "prime the pump" of procedural memory (i.e muscle memory), by the use of specific and carefully prepared materials, so that the person begins to "remember" how to wash him/herself not from the declarative memory in his head but from the procedural memory in his body.

If we do this successfully, the results could be very dramatic indeed, and may solve this difficult problem of "lack of motivation" which is the bug-bear of so many types of dementia.

2) **How to deal with "the inability to recall the steps involved in washing".**
Dr. Montessori found that another major key to success had to do with the way we lay out and present activities to a person. She learned through trial and error how to lay out activities for children in such a way that they could easily follow the steps involved. So let's take a close look at this aspect of our approach to care.

Layout and presentation of tasks.
Dr. Montessori found that when a task was broken down into segments and the materials for each segment were presented in an orderly fashion, the children became attracted to the activity and experienced success carrying out the activity from beginning to end.

Now, in our approach to older people living with dementia, we need to apply this principle of breaking down the activity into segments.

With regard to "washing", this means that we need to break down the whole process of washing into "bite-size" sections that can be presented logically.

These sections could be:

a) wheeling a carefully prepared washstand over to a person with dementia.
b) using very few words, demonstrating the pouring of a small amount of the water from the jug to the bowl.
c) replacing the jug back to a standing position.
d) lifting up the bar of soap and simulating the movements involved in rubbing it between your palms to wash your hands.
e) replacing the soap back in the soap dish.
f) indicating with a movement of your hand and a friendly smile, that it is "your turn next" to the person with dementia.

3) How to deal with "the sense of anxiety about the process of washing"

As we've stated, persons with dementia often have very specific reasons for feeling fearful and anxious about the whole process of washing. There are several things we can do to try to allay these fears.

a) Memory problems:

We need to find ways to assure the person living with dementia that if they remove their clothing to wash, they will be able to find their clothing again. A person living with dementia seems to know instinctively that, "out of sight", usually means "out of mind". This is one reason why persons with dementia seem to want every object that is important to them to to be either in their pockets, or in a bag tied on to them or in the bed beside them. They fear that if they let go of something they may not be able to remember where they put it and it may never be found again. So, they nervously and often aggressively, snatch all their possessions up into their arms and hold on to them tightly. So, how do we deal with assuring a person with dementia, that if he/she takes off their clothes to wash, these clothes won't just disappear?

Well, one way would be to build a small locker with a see-through glass door for the person to place their clothes in while they are washing.

The person could be re-assured that their clothes will remain there, in front of them while they wash.

It would be important not to allow anyone to remove this unit while the washing is taking place, even if the clothes just placed in it are dirty. Dealing with the removal of dirty clothes for washing is a whole other procedure, which often causes the greatest alarm to some people with dementia and can be a real bugbear for their carer, but the problem should be treated separately to washing. The person has enough to contend with just agreeing to washing themselves without further agreeing to having their clothes taken away to be laundered.

b) Privacy issues:

Most people with dementia are over 65 years of age. This means that many of these ladies and gents were born in the 1930s or 1940s. Morals and modesty issues were very different then to what they are now. People, in general were more modest in those times and stripping off clothes in the public view of anyone else was not common. This must be remembered when we care for someone living with dementia. If persons living with dementia are thinking as if they were back in their childhood, they would be extra diligent about being modest and private, as this was the norm during their childhood years.

We need to be very mindful of the need for privacy when helping a person living with dementia to wash. So, how can we go about assuring the person that we will protect their modesty? Well, we could use the "screens" that were popular many years ago. These were wooden screens, usually with 3 or 4 sections on hinges which a person put around themselves when they had a wash in the "scullery", or had a bath in the portable "tub" kept under the worktop in the kitchen. Using a screen may prove to be very helpful in allaying the fears of a person living with dementia that their privacy and modesty will be protected.

c) Sexual abuse:

Sexual abuse and incest were unfortunately very common in the 1930s, 40s 50s 60s and so on, partly because it was kept secret by children and adults alike and was just buried as a horrendous memory. We need to be very sensitive around issues such as undressing and washing when caring for a person living with dementia, because they may well have experienced some sort of abuse in childhood, that has been buried for many, many years, but could be brought back to the surface by bad-handling of undressing and washing issues.

So, how do we handle this potential problem? Well, we need to be non-threatening in our language and our demeanour to the person living with dementia and try to get them to do their own undressing, if they can, showing at all times that we are respectful of them and are not trying to harm them.

4) How to deal with an irrational fear of washing - ablutophobia.

Ablutophobia is an uncommon but very real fear of washing. The person with this phobia can feel nausea, anxiety, sweaty palms, headaches, rapid heart-beat, and other anxiety symptoms at the very mention of washing.
This condition is serious and should only be treated by a mental health specialist.

5) How to deal with someone's physical inability to wash themselves.

We should support any participation that the person is capable of.

Motto
"Remind me how to do things myself."

WASHING	(Indirect Approach).
Preliminary Activity:	Rubbing moisturiser on hands.
Aim:	To "jog" the person's "muscular memory" so as to re-activate the person's "subconscious ability" to perform the physical movements needed for "washing".
Motto:	"Prime the pump."

Materials:
- A small bottle of hand lotion. (non-perfumed and non-allergenic).

Procedure:
- Approach the person and greet him/her in a friendly manner.
- Sit down beside the person.
- Quietly ask, "Would you like to put some moisturiser on your hands?"
- If the answer is "yes", pour a little bit of moisturiser onto the person's palm and demonstrate with your own hands how to rub the palms of the hands together to spread the cream on, and how to rub one palm on the back of the other hand to spread the cream evenly over the hands.
- Allow the person plenty of time to rub the cream on his/her hands.
- When the person appears to be finished ask - "Are you finished?"
- If "yes", say something like - "Doesn't it make your hands feel good?"
- Next, thank the person and put away the moisturiser.
- If the person had initially said "no" to doing the activity, the best procedure would be to just squeeze a bit of moisturiser onto your own hands and, using clear and almost exaggerated movements rub the cream onto your hands making sure to rub one palm onto the back of the other hand to spread the cream evenly over both hands.
- When finished, you could say something like, "Ah, that made my hands feel really good perhaps you'd like to try it sometime". Take note of the reply.

Note:
- As a follow on activity, you could invite the person to rub moisturiser onto his/her neck, arms, legs, etc.

Motto
"Allow me to do things myself."

WASHING:	(Direct Approach).
Target Activity:	Washing one's self.
Aim:	To re-activate and "fix" into a daily routine the person's "procedural ability" to wash him/herself.
Goal:	To motivate the person to wash him/ herself regularly.

Materials:
- A washstand on castors, made at a height that can facilitate a person in a wheelchair or an armchair.
- A chair with supporting armrests that fits neatly under the washstand.
- A large but lightweight pitcher filled with warm water.
- A large ceramic bowl to hold the water.
- A bar of soap.

Note:
- These items, i.e. the pitcher and the bowl should be beautiful to look at.
- They should not be plastic but ceramic.
- They should be coloured either in pastels or they should have a pretty pattern on them.
- It is worth modelling them on pitchers and bowls that were in use in the 40's and 50's.
- The soap should be a bar of soap (not liquid soap), because liquid soap will not "jog" the muscle memory, but holding a bar of soap in the hands and rubbing the hands together until the soap produces suds, will hopefully "jog" the muscle memory and trigger an unconscious recollection of the procedures involved in washing.

D.I.Y. Hint:
A tea trolley would work very well, if it allowed room for a chair with armrests to fit underneath it.

Procedure:

- Wheel the wash stand over towards the person.
- Say "Would you like to wash your hands in this warm water?"
- If the answer is "yes", place the wash stand in front of the person's chair.
- Lift the pitcher and pour a little water into the bowl.
- Replace the pitcher to a standing position.
- Indicate to the person with a gesture of your hand that it's now his/her turn to do the same.
- Allow the person plenty of time to pour water from the pitcher to the bowl.
- Now, lift up the bar of soap and say "soap".
- Now place the bar of soap back in the soap dish.
- Indicate to the person with a gesture of your hand that it's now his/her turn to take up the soap.
- Allow the person plenty of time to register the message that he/she needs to lift up the soap.
- Then wait to see if he/she automatically remembers how to rub the soap onto his/her hands to produce suds.
- If the person appears not to know what to do with the bar of soap, just simulate with your two hands the movements made in the preliminary activity.
- Don't speak while you are doing the simulation, let the person concentrate on your hands, not on your speech.
- Keep doing this simulation, until the person starts to copy you.
- Leave him/her washing hands without interruption for up to ten minutes.
- When the person is finished, point to the towel and say "towel".
- Allow the person to reach over and take the towel to dry his/her hands.
- If the person still does not reach for the towel, reach for it yourself, and offer it to the person saying, "here's the towel to dry your hands".
- When the hands are dry, indicate with your finger the hook for the towel to be hung back on.
- Allow the person time to register what you mean, and time to carry out the action.
- If the person does not attempt to hang the towel up, hang it up yourself saying "I'll just hang up the towel".
- Finally, smile and say "Are you finished washing your hands?"
- If "yes", thank the person and take away the wash stand.

Note:

- Gradually extend this activity to include washing face, neck, arms, torso, etc.
- Do not try to do all of this on the first sitting.

DRESSING

Things To Ponder

Most people living with dementia have probably buttoned and unbuttoned shirts, fastened and unfastened cardigans, zipped and unzipped jackets/jumpers and trousers, thousands of times throughout their lives. But now, a combination of difficulties has turned these everyday dressing activities into daunting or even impossible tasks.

The difficulties involved are:

Mental Confusion.
The person living with dementia is often confused about the function of the particular piece of clothing. They may mistake a jumper for a pair of trousers and spent an inordinate amount of time trying to put their feet into an arm-hole and so on, often losing their balance in the process. This confusion is usually caused by damage to the semantic memory which helps us to remember the functions of things.

Visual Confusion.
The confusion could also be caused by visual-perception problems which people with dementia frequently experience, whereby they don't see things properly and therefore can't work out what they are.

Dexterity Problems.
People with dementia are frequently aged and therefore may have additional problems such as arthritis in the fingers, which makes opening and closing buttons and other fastenings a very difficult activity indeed.

The Good News

If the person living with dementia is given opportunities to practice these skills regularly in an orderly and tranquil fashion, there is a good chance that his/her muscular memory will be re-activated and, within time, he/she will be able to open and close buttons, fasten and unfasten belts and do undo zips once again. So, let's examine how we can "remind" a person living with dementia how to perform a skill that was once second nature to them, i.e. dressing one's self.

Motto
"Remind me how to do things myself."

DRESSING	(Indirect Approach).
Preliminary Activity:	Using dressing frames.
Aim:	To "jog" the person's "muscular memory" so as to re-activate the person's "subconscious ability" to perform the physical actions involved in "dressing."
Motto:	"Prime the pump."

Materials:
- A trolley on castors.
- Individual dressing frames, such as:
- A button frame, a buckle frame, a zip frame or a snap frame.

Procedure:
- Take the trolley on which is placed one dressing frame only.
- Approach the person in a friendly manner and greet him/her.
- Ask, "Would you like me to show you this button frame?"
- If "yes", sit next to the person on his/her dominant side.
- Hold the button frame with both hands and allow the person to view it.
- Then slowly, with exaggerated movements, start to open the top button.
- When you've opened one or two buttons, indicate to the person with a hand gesture that he/she may have a turn.
- Allow the person plenty of time to open a button.
- Encourage the person to open the next button and the one after it.
- When all the buttons have been opened, smile and say, "Now I suppose we have to close them again."
- Close the top button yourself.
- Now gesture to the person to close the next button and the next until all the buttons have been closed.
- Finally, thank the person for his/her participation. Arrange to do it again.

Motto
"Allow me to do things myself"

DRESSING   (Direct Approach).

Target Activity: **Dressing one's self.**

Aim: To re-activate and "fix" into a daily routine the person's "procedural ability" to dress him/herself.

Goal: To motivate the person to dress him/herself daily.

Materials:
- A clothes rail on castors, fixed to a height that makes it possible for a person in a wheelchair or armchair to reach it and lift off an item of clothing.
- 3 items of clothing, each on a separate hanger. These should be arranged logically e.g. a blouse/shirt, a cardigan/jumper, a skirt/trousers.

Procedure:
- Wheel the trolley over towards the person who may be in a wheelchair.
- Ask politely, "Would you like to get dressed?"
- If the answer is "no" leave the trolley standing there for a while in the hope that the person will become interested.
- If the answer is "yes", proceed as follows:
- Lift the hanger holding the blouse (this should be the first item on the rail).
- Show it to the person saying "Would you like to wear this lovely blouse/shirt?
- Presuming the person says "yes", hold the blouse in the view of the person with your non-dominant hand and with your dominant hand, aid the person to remove their pyjama top or whatever clothing needs to be removed so that he/she can put on the blouse.
- Keep the blouse/shirt in the person's sight all the time, because when one has dementia, "out of sight" usually means "out of mind", so the person needs to see the blouse/shirt all the time so that he/she is reminded that the taking off of the pyjama top is necessary so that he/she can put on the blouse/shirt.
- Allow the person to take the blouse/shirt off the hanger him/herself if he/she is able to, only give help if needed.

- Do not request that the person puts the hanger back on the rail yet, this is a separate activity which can be done when the dressing is complete. To do this now will distract the person from focusing on dressing, which is the point of this activity.
- Allow the person time to examine the blouse/shirt. He/she may start to count the buttons or start trying to fasten up the button holes. Do not interfere with this activity but try to get the focus back on dressing by saying "Would you like to put your blouse/shirt on?"
- If the person says "yes", then be ready to offer assistance, but only give assistance if really needed.
- When the blouse/shirt is on, point to the buttons saying something like "Oh, what a lot of buttons, would you like to fasten them?"
- Allow the person time to think about this.
- If the person does not begin to fasten the button, offer to fasten one for him/her, making sure to do this using very little speech and clear and exaggerated movements.
- Indicate by a hand movement that it is the person's turn to fasten the next button and the next etc.
- When all the buttons are fastened (or as many as the person wishes to do), say something like: "You look very well in that blouse/shirt. The colour suits you."
- Repeat this approach with the skirt/trousers, only offering help if needed or required.
- Finally, when the person is dressed, say something like, "You look wonderful to-day."
- Then take the trolley with the empty hangers away.
- You could invite the person to help you to put the hangers back on the rail, if he/she wanted to.
- Finally, thank the person for his/her participation and ask if he/she would like to do the same tomorrow.

Self-Esteem.

Being able to dress one's self gives a feeling of independence to a person of any age and a feeling of independence leads to a feeling of high self-esteem, which in itself is a morale booster.

What this means, in effect, is that, regular positive experiences, such as successfully dressing oneself will bring about a more positive mind-set in a person living with dementia.

Dr. Montessori proved, in her work with children, that physical activities have a direct link to the emotional and psychological well-being of the human being. Regular opportunities to carry out physical activities such as putting on your shirt yourself, buttoning your cardigan yourself, slipping on your shoes yourself and so on may not seem like very significant activities to the person who does not have dementia, but to the person who does have this condition, carrying out these activities successfully has great significance. It tells the person that they are not useless, they are not dependent, they are not childish, they are not a burden on everyone else.

These are the things that are of huge significance to the human spirit in every person. We all have a human need to feel worthwhile and being able to dress ourselves independently is a major step in helping a person with dementia to feel "worthwhile".

GROOMING

Things To Ponder

Combing your hair, shaving, clipping your nails, are all aspects of good grooming. Most people living with dementia have done these things for years and years. Now, however, the disability has interfered with their recollection of how and when to do these things.

The Good News

Combing hair, shaving and other grooming tasks are done by way of "muscle memory". Most of us can comb our hair with our eyes closed. We have ingrained the actions into our "muscle memory". This means that when a person with dementia has "forgotten" how and when to do these things, we may be able to re-activate the "muscular memory" of how to do these things by getting the person to carry out very precise activities designed to "jog" that muscle memory.

Motto
"Remind me how to do things myself."

GROOMING	(Indirect Approach).
Preliminary Activity:	Combing hair on a styling head. (D.I.Y. hint: use a Barbie Doll S/Head).
Aim:	To "jog" the person's "muscular memory" so as to re-activate the person's "subconscious ability" to perform the physical actions involved in combing hair.
Motto:	"Prime the pump".

Materials:
- A trolley on castors, on which is placed:-
- A styling head with a wig on it, (a long wig for ladies, a short wig for gents).
- A wide-toothed comb.

Procedure:
- Wheel the trolley over near the person.
- Approach the person in a friendly manner and greet him/her.
- Ask, "Would you like to help me to comb this hair?"
- If "yes", sit beside the person (to his/her dominant side).
- Lift up the comb and slowly and deliberately start to comb the hair on the styling head from the top to the bottom.
- After a few strokes say "Would you like to have a go?"
- Allow the person plenty of time to comb the hair.
- Encourage long strokes from the top of the head to the bottom of the hair strands.
- When the person has had enough say, "Wow, that hair looks great!"
- Remove the trolley and thank the person for his/her participation.

Extensions to this activity: (for ladies).
- curling the hair with hair rollers.
- plaiting the hair, putting pony-tails in the hair, putting hair grips in the hair.

Motto
"Allow me to do things myself."

GROOMING   (Direct Approach).

Target Activity: Combing one's hair.

Aim: To re-activate and "fix" into a daily routine the person's "procedural ability" to comb his/her hair.

Goal: To motivate the person to groom him/herself regularly.

Materials:
- A trolley on castors.
- A tray.
- A wide-toothed comb.
- A hand mirror.
- A template sheet with a silhouette of a comb and a hand-mirror printed on it.

Procedure:
- Wheel the trolley over to the person.
- Greet the person in a dignified but friendly manner. Introduce yourself.
- Quietly ask, "Would you like to comb your hair?"
- If "yes", lift up the comb, say, "Here's the comb", then put the comb on the tray.
- Indicate, with a hand gesture, that it is the person's turn to take up the comb.
- Allow the person plenty of time to register what you are saying.
- If nothing happens, repeat the previous two steps.
- When the person lifts up the comb, simulate a combing gesture on your own hair, just to "prime the pump" of procedural memory.
- When the person has finished combing his/her hair, indicate by pointing with your finger, that the comb needs to be replaced onto the template on the tray.
- Finally, lift up the hand-mirror and say, "Here's the mirror".
- Then replace the mirror onto the template on the tray .
- Indicate, by pointing your with your finger and using a hand gesture that the person is welcome to lift up the mirror and use it.
- Allow the person plenty of time to register this next step.
- When the person is finished using the mirror, say "Wow, you look wonderful".
- Remove the trolley and thank the person.

EATING

Things To Ponder

Most persons living with dementia have been using spoons, knives and forks, or chop-sticks to feed themselves for over 50 or 60 years. But now, because of this illness, they often become confused about how to get food from the plate or the bowl into their mouths. The reasons for this confusion are many. One reason for the confusion has to do with semantic memory, i.e the part of memory that reminds us what the functions and purposes of things are. Semantic memory, when it's working properly, tells us things like, "that's a spoon, you use it to scoop up your cornflakes", or "that's a fork, you use it to lift your fries to your mouth", or "that's a knife, you use it to cut up your food". Semantic memory does this in microseconds, so we are never consciously aware of how we remember the functions of things. It is only when we notice that someone can no longer remember the purpose of a knife, fork or spoon that we become aware that something very strange is happening to his/her memory. To an observer, this often looks like an irreversible problem, but it isn't.

The Good News

When we lift up a knife, fork or spoon and start to bring it towards our mouth, we are actually making use of the part of memory called "procedural" or "muscle" memory. This means we don't need to think about every step in the procedure. The procedure just "flows" from one muscle movement to another.

This is precisely the part of memory we need to re-activate in the person living with dementia, who now suffers damage to his/her semantic memory.

Even persons in their eighties, living with dementia can be helped to regain the "habit" of feeding themselves with a utensil such as a spoon, knife, fork, chop-sticks or their fingers, as is the habit in some cultures, by the re-activation of "procedural memory". Regaining this "habit" will involve two things,- firstly, the use of indirect activities which will prepare the person for the target activity, i.e eating with a utensil and secondly, the use of repetition of the task to ingrain the procedure in the person's "muscle memory".

So, let's see how we might go about achieving this.

Motto
"Remind me how to do things myself."

EATING   (Indirect Approach).

Preliminary Activity: Scooping sweets from a bowl of rice.

Aim: To "jog" the person's "muscular
                                          memory", so as to re-activate the
                                          person's "subconscious ability" to
                                          perform the physical actions involved
                                          in manipulating a feeding utensil.

Motto: "Prime the pump."

Materials:
- A trolley on which is placed a tray holding:
- 2 bowls, one large and one small.
- A bag of white uncooked rice.
- 8 soft sweets such as maltezers.
- A sieve spoon with holes large enough for the rice to escape from it

Procedure:
- Wheel the trolley with the tray on it over towards the person.
- Greet the person in a friendly manner and introduce yourself.
- Sit next to the person (on his/her dominant side).
- Ask, "May I show you this bowl of rice?"
- If "yes", slowly and deliberately lift the sieve spoon and scoop up some rice.
- Let the rice fall through the holes, in full view of the person.
- Keep scooping up spoonfuls of rice until you scoop up a maltezer.
- When you do manage to scoop up a maltezer take it out of the sieve spoon and place it in the small round bowl. Now offer the person a turn to do the same.
- Each time the person scoops up a maltezer, indicate that it must be put in the bowl.
- When the 8 sweets have been scooped up and placed in the bowl, the activity is finished.
- Finally, invite the person to eat the sweets with you or share them with others.

Note: This activity has a useful intergenerational aspect to it. It would be a very enjoyable game for a person to play with a grandchild or a child visitor.

Motto
"Allow me to do things myself."

EATING	(Direct Approach).
Target Activity:	Feeding one's self.
Aim:	To re-activate and "fix" into a daily routine the person's "procedural ability" to manipulate a feeding utensil again.
Goal:	To motivate the person to feed him/herself daily.

Materials:
- A trolly on castors containing:
- A tray.
- A bowl of porridge.
- A spoon.

Procedure:
- Wheel the trolley over towards the person and greet him/her in a friendly way.
- Sit beside the person (to his/her dominant side), and introduce yourself.
- Say, "I've brought you a lovely bowl of porridge." Ask, "Are you hungry?"
- If "yes", lift the tray with the bowl of porridge on it and place it on a table in front of the person or on the person's lap, supporting it with your left hand.
- Encourage the person to lift the spoon and scoop up the porridge as in the preliminary activity.
- If the person doesn't do this, put your right hand under his/her elbow and guide the person's arm and hand to perform a scooping motion.
- When spooning begins, try not to distract the person by talking, allow him/her to focus on spooning food into his/her mouth.
- Allow the person plenty of time to spoon the food into his/her mouth.
- When the person is finished, say "That was lovely porridge, did you enjoy it?"
- Remove the tray and place it back on the trolley.
- Offer the person a cup of tea and if possible sit and chat with the person.
- When you are both finished the tea, say, "I have to go now but would you like me to bring you a bowl of porridge again tomorrow?" Take note of the reply.
- Finally, remove the trolly.

TOILETING

Things To Ponder

The average lady or gentleman living with dementia will have been using a toilet independently for over 60 years. It is even possible that he/she may have changed the nappies of the person now caring for them, if that person is a son or daughter. But now, things have changed and it seems like the child is father of the man or mother of the woman, so to speak. This situation necessarily causes problems.

Many elderly people living with dementia develop incontinence. This often occurs suddenly after an acute illness when the person becomes bed-ridden for some time and is too ill to stand up go to the toilet and of necessity has to use incontinence pads. Other times, incontinence occurs gradually, especially with certain types of dementia, in particular those which involve mini-strokes. Incontinence causes a new habit to form, the habit of passing urine directly into a pad rather than a toilet. Our job then is to help the person to try to break this new habit of passing urine directly into a pad and regain the habit of using the toilet.

The Good News

This job is not as hard as you might imagine. Many people, even those in their eighties can be helped to get back into the "habit" of using a toilet, but the task demands persistence and consistency.

We can personally attest that even persons in late stage dementia can be helped to regain continence (even if only during the waking hours), by "priming the pump" of procedural memory.

Remember, habits are formed through repetitive, consistent behaviour, so our task in ending the habit of incontinence and regaining continence, will require repetitive, consistent, behaviour.

Initially, the person will need a third party, i.e. a carer or family member to continuously invite them to use the toilet, but after a few days of these constant reminders, the person will usually start to initiate going to the toilet themselves. This can seem miraculous in people who have been "incontinent" for a long period, but it isn't really miraculous at all, it is the brain beginning to use "muscle memory" again.

TOILETING	(Indirect Approach).
Preliminary Activity:	Using a commode.
Aim:	To "jog" the person's "muscular memory" so as to re-activate the person's "subconscious ability" to perform the physical actions involved in using a commode/toilet once again.
Motto:	"Prime the pump."

Materials:
- A commode.
- A roll of toilet paper.
- Some hand-wipes (antibacterial).
- A screen.

Procedure:
- Approach the person in a quite and dignified manner.
- Quietly ask the person if he/she needs to use a commode.
- If the person says "no", don't persist. Say, "I'll check with you later."
- If the person says "yes", place a screen around the person and discretely wheel in a commode for the person's use.
- Help the person to sit on the commode, being careful all the time to preserve the person's dignity.
- When the person appears to be finished, offer him/her the toilet roll, once again using a quiet voice, preserving the person's privacy and dignity.
- Now offer the person some antibacterial hand- wipes.
- Help the person back into bed or into a chair and thank him/her.
- Remove the commode and wash it.
- Repeat this procedure several times a day.
- When you think the person might be ready to use a toilet, move on to the target activity, using a toilet.

Motto
"Help me to preserve my dignity."

TOILETING	(Direct Approach).
Target Activity:	Using a toilet.
Aim:	To re-activate and "fix" into a routine the person's "procedural ability" to use a toilet.
Goal:	To motivate the person to use the toilet regularly again.

Materials:
- A toilet.

(There should be no clutter in the toilet room. Take everything that is portable out of the room, because extra items in the room may cause confusion to the person with dementia).

Procedure:
- Approach the person in a pleasant manner and ask in a very quiet voice, "Would you like me to show you where the toilet is?" or "Would you like me to help you to go into the toilet?"
- If the person says "no", don't persist, say "that's fine, I'll check with you later, call me if you need me." This hopefully will plant the thought in the person's head that they might need the toilet later.
- Ten minutes later, repeat this.
- Ten minutes later, repeat this again.
- Keep repeating until the answer is "yes".
- When the person says "yes", kindly help him/her, to go into the toilet room.
- If the person is wet, remove the wet pad in a gentle and dignified fashion but make sure to get the person to sit on the toilet while you're doing this.
- Remember, it is the habit of sitting on the toilet we want to revive, so it is imperative that the person sits on the toilet regularly even if he/she does not feel the urge to use it.
- While the person is sitting on the toilet, help him/her to put on a clean pad.
- If the person is not wet, all the better, allow him/her time to sit on the toilet until he/she feels the flow of water or other matter.
- When the person appears to be finished, ask "Are you finished? If "yes" allow him/her time to pull up the pad him/herself, only give help if requested.

CARE OF ONE'S ENVIRONMENT

Activities for Ladies.
- Pegging Clothes.
- Folding Laundry.

Activities for Gents.
- Watering Plants.
- Washing Windows.

CARE OF ONE'S ENVIRONMENT

Things To Ponder

A very real problem encountered by people living with dementia is that they gradually lose interest in caring for their own immediate environment.

Ladies, who spent many years doing daily tasks such as washing dishes, sweeping floors, pegging up laundry, setting the table for family dinners, now seem to have no memory of, nor interest in, doing, these tasks.

Gents, who spent many years doing such tasks as watering the garden, fixing appliances, putting nuts on bolts, using hammers and nails, now also seem to have no memory of, nor interest in, doing, these tasks.

As a result of this lack of interest, everyone assumes that the person living with dementia can't do these things anymore. Family members, so distraught at their loved one's diagnosis of dementia, try to help by doing everything for the person. We visit our loved one's home and we wash the dishes, we sweep the floor, we set the table, we water the grass, we fix the broken appliances. We assume, the whole time, that our loved one will never be able to do these things again.

But, that's where we are wrong.

The Good News.

Even people with advanced dementia can still do some things . We may just have to "prime the pump" of "muscle memory" to get the flow going once again.

What we need to be aware of, all the time is, that every human being needs to do meaningful activity i.e "work", everyday of their lives. If someone else does everything for us then we have no logical reason to wake up in the mornings, and probably no motivation to get out of bed either.

Having something to look forward to motivates us to want to get out of bed in the morning. This could be a simple thing like looking forward to weeding that vegetable patch, or looking forward to tidying out that larder.

Whatever the task is, it gives meaning and purpose to someone's life, and it is our job to try to support it.

Motto
"Remind me how to care for my own environment."

PEGGING	(Indirect Approach).
Preliminary Activity:	Putting clothes pegs around a bowl.
Aim:	To "jog" the person's "muscular memory" so as to re-activate the person's "subconscious ability" to perform the physical actions involved in opening and closing pegs.
Motto:	"Prime the pump."

Materials:
- A tray.
- A bowl.
- 10 clothes pegs.

Procedure:
- Approach the person in a friendly manner.
- Greet the person and introduce yourself.
- Ask "Could I show you this job I'm doing?"
- If the person says "yes", proceed as follows:
- Using very slow and deliberate actions, between your thumb and forefinger, lift up a peg and squeeze until the peg opens.
- Put the peg on the rim of the bowl.
- Repeat.
- After you have pegged about 2 or 3 pegs onto the rim of the bowl, indicate with a gesture of your hand that it is the person's turn to place a peg on the rim of the bowl.
- Allow the person plenty of time to pick up a peg, squeeze it between their thumb and forefinger and peg it onto the rim of the bowl.
- Encourage the person to do the same with the next peg and the next until all the pegs are on the rim of the bowl.
- When all the pegs are on the rim of the bowl say something like-"That's great".
- Inquire if the person enjoyed the activity and if he/she would like to repeat it.
- Finally, thank the person for their co-operation.

Motto
"Allow me to care for my own environment."

PEGGING	(Direct Approach).
Target Activity:	Pegging clothes onto a low line.
Aim:	To re-activate and "fix" into a routine the person's "procedural ability" to peg wet clothes onto a low line.
Goal:	To motivate the person to start caring for their own environment again by taking responsibility for their wet clothes and hanging them up to dry.

Materials:
- A small basket containing 6 small wet items which need to be hung on a line.
- A small basket containing 12 clothes pegs.
- An indoor/outdoor portable clothes line, made at a height that makes it accessible to persons who are seated in an armchair or a wheelchair.

Procedure:
- Approach the person in a friendly fashion and greet him/her.
- Say "Please could you help me to hang some wet clothes on the line?'
- If "yes", reach into the basket and take out 1 item of laundry, e.g. a face flannel.
- Reach into the peg bowl and take out a peg.
- Slowly and deliberately hold the face flannel up to the line and put a peg in the left corner.
- Reach into the peg basket and select another peg.
- Slowly and deliberately, put the second peg onto the right corner of the flannel to hold it in place.
- With a gesture of your hand, indicate to the person that it is their turn to peg an item of clothing /laundry onto the line.
- Allow the person plenty of time to peg up an item.
- Encourage the person to hang up the others until they are all hung up.
- When all the items are hung up say to the person something like "wow, you've done a great job!"
- Leave the items to dry on the line.
- Thank the person for their co-operation.

Motto
"Remind me how to care for my own environment."

FOLDING   (Indirect Approach).

Preliminary Activity: Creasing a napkin.

Aim: To "jog" the person's "muscular memory" so as to re-activate the person's "subconscious ability" to perform the physical actions involved in "folding" something over on itself and creasing it.

Motto: "Prime the pump."

Materials:
- A trolley containing:
- A tray.
- Table napkins with a dotted line drawn on each of them to indicate where to put a crease.

Procedure:
- Approach the person in a friendly manner and greet him/her.
- Sit at the person's dominant side and introduce yourself.
- Ask, "Please, would you help me to fold these napkins.
- If "yes", proceed as follows:
- Select one napkin.
- Spread the napkin out on the tray.
- Slowly and deliberately, run your forefinger over the dotted line.
- Next, hold the left and right end corners of the napkin between the thumb and forefinger of your left and right hands.
- Fold the napkin over on itself.
- Crease the napkin by pressing on the folded area.
- With a gesture of your hand, indicate to the person that it is their turn to fold a napkin.
- Allow the person plenty of time to select and fold a napkin.
- Encourage the person to fold another and another.
- When all the napkins are folded, say, "wow, what a great job you've done".
- Thank the person, and remove the trolley.

Motto
"Allow me to care for my own environment."

FOLDING   (Direct Approach).

Target Activity: Folding Laundry.

Aim: To re-activate and "fix" into a daily routine the person's "procedural ability" to "fold" their own clothes.

Goal: To motivate the person to fold their own clothes and put them away tidily.

Materials:
- A trolley.
- A laundry basket containing clean laundry.
- A tray.

Procedure:
- Approach the person in a friendly manner and greet him/her.
- Sit beside the person to their dominant side and introduce yourself.
- Ask, "please would you help me to fold this laundry?"
- If "yes", proceed as follows:
- Take out an item of laundry from the basket.
- Spread it out on the trolley.
- Hold the item using the thumb and forefinger of your left and right hands.
- Fold the cloth over on itself.
- Fold again, if necessary.
- When the item is folded neatly, place it in the tray.
- Now, indicate to the person that it is his/her turn to fold an item of laundry.
- Allow the person plenty of time to select and fold an item of laundry.
- When an item is folded and placed on the tray, encourage the person to fold another and another.
- Continue in this manner until all the items are folded.
- Try not to talk, as this may distract the person and cause confusion.
- When all the items have been folded, say something like, "great job!".
- Ask the person if he/she enjoyed the task and if he/she would like to do it again some other day.
- Finally, thank the person and put the trolley away.

Motto
"Remind me how to care for my own environment."

WATERING PLANTS	(Indirect Approach).
Preliminary Activity:	Pouring water from jug to jug.
Aim:	To "jog" the person's "muscular memory" so as to re-activate the person's "subconscious ability" to perform the physical actions involved in holding a jug and tilting it over to release the water from it.
Motto:	"Prime the pump."

Materials:
- A trolley on which is placed:
- A tray containing:
- 2 small jugs, one half full of water.
- A sponge to mop up spills.

Procedure:
- (First ascertain whether the person is right or left handed).
- Approach the person in a friendly manner and greet him.
- Sit beside the person to his dominant side and introduce yourself.
- Ask, "Could I show you something?"
- If "yes", place the tray containing the jugs and sponge either on a table in front of the person, (who may be in a wheelchair), or on the person's lap, if he/she is in bed.
- Assuming you are seated to the right of the person, slowly and deliberately, lift the jug with your right hand, supporting the bottom of the jug with your left hand, and pour the water carefully from the jug into the other jug on the tray.
- (Reverse this if the person is left-handed).
- When you've done that, pause for a moment, and then reverse the positions of the jug, so that the jug containing the water is on the right again.
- Now, indicate to the person that it is his turn to pour from jug to jug.
- Allow the person plenty of time and do not make a fuss if the water spills, just mop it up quietly and discretely.

- Encourage the person to repeat the procedure over and over, as he/she will get better at it with practice.
- When the person is clearly finished, show him/her how to mop up the spills with the sponge.
- Now, thank the person for his/her co-operation and ask if he/she would like to do the activity again some other time.
- Lastly, put away the materials.

Motto
"Allow me to care for my own environment."

WATERING PLANTS   (Direct Approach).

Target Activity: Watering Plants and Flowers.

Aim: To re-activate and "fix" into a routine the person's "procedural ability" to "water the plants".

Goal: To motivate the person to engage in meaningful activity i.e "work" and to take an interest in caring for his/her own environment by watering the plants.

Materials:
- A trolley on castors on which is placed:
- A tray that will sit neatly on a person's lap or on a small table.
- 6 potted plants in small to medium sized pots, (all of which look a bit different in either colour, size or shape of foliage).
- A watering can containing just enough water for one plant.
- A bottle of water for refilling the watering can.
- A sponge for mopping up spills.

Procedure:
- Approach the person in a friendly manner and greet him.
- Ask, "Could you help me to water these plants?"
- If "yes", place the tray on the table (or lap, holding one side to keep it steady).
- Place one plant only on the tray.
- Next, lift the watering can off the trolley and place it on the tray.
- Say, "This is the watering can".
- Next, (assuming you are sitting to the right of the person), with your right hand lift up the watering can and pour a little water on the plant.
- Then place the can down on the tray.
- Now indicate to the person that it is his turn to do the same.
- Allow the person time to grasp what he has to do.
- Observe closely as he tilts the watering can. Try not to interfere or talk.
- When the plant is watered, lift it off the tray and place it on the lower shelf of the trolley.

- Now, put the second plant on the person's tray.
- Refill the watering can from the bottle, putting in just enough water to hydrate one plant.
- Place the watering can on the person's tray.
- Indicate with a gesture that it is the person's turn to water the plant.
- When the plant is watered, lift it off the tray, as before, and place it on the lower shelf of the trolley.
- Now, put the third plant on the person's tray.
- Repeat this procedure until all 6 plants have been watered.
- When all 6 plants are watered and are placed on the lower shelf of the trolley, say something like, "Well done, the plants are all watered now".
- Take a few minutes to admire the plants with the person.
- If the person initiates a conversation about flowers or plants, be ready to encourage it, this may lead to reminiscence about the person's own garden or their memories of watering flowers in childhood. Always be ready for a gem of recollection to emerge.
- Finally, thank the person for their help.

WASHING WINDOWS   (Indirect Approach).

Preliminary Activity: Cleaning a Mirror

Aim: To "jog" the person's "muscular memory" so as to re-activate the person's "subconscious ability" to perform the physical actions needed to wash glass.

Motto: "Prime the pump"

Goal: To motivate the person to engage in meaningful activity, i.e "work".

Materials:
- A trolley on castors containing:
- A tray.
- A hand mirror.
- 2 small cleaning cloths.
- A small bottle with a spray top containing water with lemon and vinegar in it.

Procedure:
- Approach the person who may be sitting down or in a wheel-chair.
- Greet the person in a friendly but dignified manner and introduce yourself.
- Ask, "Would you like to see what I have here?"
- If "yes", take the tray off the trolley and place it on your lap.
- Say, "This is a mirror and I'm going to clean it, would you help me please?"
- If "yes", hand one cleaning cloth to the person and take the other cleaning cloth yourself.
- With your left hand, spray a bit of the water /vinegar /lemon on to the mirror.
- With your right hand, start to wipe the surface of the mirror.
- Indicate to the person that he/she should now wipe the mirror with a cloth.
- Wipe together until the mirror is clean, spraying the water as needed.
- Offer the person an opportunity to spray the water also.
- When the mirror is clean, say, "Well, didn't we do a great job."
- Thank the person for his/her help.
- Ask the person if he/she would like to do this again sometime.

Motto
"Allow me to care for my own environment".

WASHING WINDOWS   (Direct Approach).

Target Activity: Cleaning windows

Aim: To re-activate and fix into a routine the person's "procedural ability" to wash windows.

Goal: To motivate the person to engage in meaningful activity, i.e. "work".

Materials:
- A trolley on castors containing:
- 2 window wipers.
- 2 bottles with spray tops containing water with a little vinegar and lemon.

Procedure:
- Approach the person in a friendly manner and introduce yourself.
- Sit beside the person (to his/her dominant side).
- Say, "I'm going to wash the windows, would you like to help me?"
- If "yes", say, "here's your window wiper", as you place the wiper in his/her hand.
- Either wheel the person, if he/she is in a wheelchair, or walk with the person over to the window that needs washing.
- Make sure to remove all items from the window sill that could be in the way, or could be a distraction to the person, i.e plants or ornaments.
- Now, taking your spay bottle in your left hand, spray a little water on the window.
- As the water rolls down the window, using your right hand, use the window wiper to clean the window.
- Indicate to the person to do the same.
- Continue spraying and wiping together until the window is clean.
- When finished, say, "Well, this window is really clean now, we did a great job."
- If the person appears to have enjoyed the activity, ask, "Would you like to help me to wash another window?"
- If "yes", repeat as above. If "no", say, "Maybe another time then".
- Finally, thank the person for his/her help and, if possible, sit and chat with the person for a while. Maybe a conversation will begin about who used to do the "window washing" in his/her home in times past. Be ready, enjoy the moment.

CARE OF OTHERS

- Laying a Table for a Meal
- Polishing Shoes for Others.

CARE OF OTHERS

Things To Ponder.

When people are living with dementia either at home or in residential care, we often assume that they are not capable of, or interested in, the welfare of others. This is not actually true at all. We once witnessed a person in late stage dementia almost running with her zimmer frame in an effort to give another resident a handkerchief that had fallen from his pocket,

Many times, we have seen residents in nursing homes walking around the communal room sharing sweets that some friend had given them with other residents, or trying to help another resident to stand up or put on their slippers.

There is something in the heart of most human beings that urges them to reach out to others in order to care or share. A person may only wish to share with one trusted friend or a person may reach out to a group, but, the instinct is still the same. Most human beings feel an instinct to take an interest in the welfare of others.

The Good News.

When a person living with dementia is given opportunities to do something for others, he/she begins to feel valued and useful once again. Dr. Montessori wrote:

"feeling one's own value, being appreciated and loved by others, feeling useful and capable of production are all factors of enormous value for the human soul".

Because this instinct to reach out to others is present in most people, our task is not to create it, but merely to resurrect it. The good news is that we can usually do this by engaging the person with dementia in carefully planned out everyday activities which involve doing something for others. These activities should not be new or foreign to the person, but should be ordinary activities that the person has done hundreds of times in their lives without consciously thinking about them.

Two such activities are: setting a table for a meal, which was traditionally carried out by ladies, and, polishing shoes for oneself and others, which was traditionally carried out by gents.

SETTING A TABLE FOR A MEAL

Things To Ponder.

Most ladies living with dementia will have spent many, many years setting the table for family meals. This would have involved a series of actions that they did automatically, e.g laying out placemats, laying out knives, forks and spoons, laying out drinking glasses, cups and saucers, or even a candlestick or vase of flowers.

The task was both practical and aesthetic and gave the person a feeling of satisfaction when she stood back and gave a quick glance over the table to see if everything was in the correct position.

Most older ladies would tell you that they could set a table with their eyes closed. Now, however, since the onset of dementia, many people cannot remember these steps.

The Good News

Since setting a table for a meal involves steps held in the "muscle memory". carefully devised activities may help the person with dementia to re-activate that "muscle memory" so that, once again, the person can set the table for a family meal and by doing so, feel useful again and feel that she is making a contribution to others.

Making a contribution enhances self-esteem. Enhanced self-esteem results in less anxiety and depression. Less anxiety and depression results in more positive behaviour and so a cycle of positivity begins.

If we can achieve all this by helping a person to remember how to set a table for a meal, we will have achieved something great indeed.

Motto
"Remind me how to do things for others."

SETTING A TABLE   (Indirect Approach).

Preliminary Activity: Matching plates and cutlery to silhuettes on a template.

Aim: To "jog" the person's "muscular memory" so as to re-activate the person's "subconscious ability" to perform the physical actions involved in setting a table for a meal.

Motto: "Prime the pump."

Materials:
• A trolley on castors on which is placed:
• A specially made laminated table mat template on which is drawn a silhouette of a plate, a knife, a fork and a spoon.
• An adult sized dinner plate, knife, fork and spoon.

Procedure:
• Approach the person in a friendly manner and greet him/her.
• Ask, "Could I show you something I made?"
• Pulling the trolley over near you and the person, lift up the laminated mat and show it to the person. Point to the silhouette of the plate, then the silhouette of the knife, fork and spoon. Now, place the mat back on the tray.
• Slowly and deliberately, and preferably with no speech, lift the plate and place it on the silhouette of the plate.
• Now slowly and deliberately, and with no speech, lift the knife and place it on the silhouette of the knife.
• Now, slowly and deliberately, and with no speech, lift the fork and place it on the silhouette of the fork.
• Lastly, slowly and deliberately, and with no speech, lift the spoon and place it on the silhouette of the spoon.
• Now, sit back and look approvingly at what you've done.
• Then, slowly and deliberately, and preferably with no speech, lift off the plate, then the knife, then the fork, and spoon and place them back on the trolley.
• Now offer the person a turn and follow the exact same procedure.
• When the person is finished, remember to thank him/her for their help.

Motto
"Invite me to do things for others."

SETTING A TABLE	(Direct Approach).
Target Activity:	Setting a table for a meal.
Aim:	To re-activate and "fix" into a routine the person's "procedural ability" to set a table for a meal.
Goal:	To encourage the person to do things for others, so as to help them to feel a sense of their own worth and value.

Materials:
- A table, preferably rectangular, on which is placed a clear white table cloth with no patterns.
- A trolley on castors containing:
- 4 dinner plates.
- 4 knifes.
- 4 forks.
- 4 spoons.

Procedure:
- Approach the person in a friendly manner and greet her.
- Ask, "Could you help me to set a table for dinner?"
- If "yes", take the person with you to the table, where you have left the prepared trolley.
- Say, "We need to put four plates on the table".
- Allow the person time to register what needs to be done.
- Hand a plate to the person and say, "Could you put that plate on the table please".
- Hand the next plate to the person giving the same instruction.
- Continue until all 4 plates are on the table.
- Now say, "Could you put a knife and fork beside each plate please".
- Hand a knife and fork to the person.
- Guide the person, if needed, if there's confusion, just give one item at a time.
- Try not to talk too much as talk may confuse the person.
- When all the cutlery has been laid out on the table, stand back and, with great enthusiasm say, "Well, doesn't this look lovely. You did a great job".
- Thank the lady for helping and ask if she would like to do it again sometime.

POLISHING SHOES

Things To Ponder

Most gentlemen living with dementia, are over 75 years of age. This means that they were born in the 1940's or earlier. Now, during those years, men's shoes were always made of leather and there was only one way to keep them clean - polish them.

Polishing shoes was a daily activity. Many men polished their shoes the night before work. It was often their last job before turning out the light. I remember my father used to get us all to leave our shoes by the fireplace on a Saturday evening so he could polish them and have them all looking spick and span for church on Sunday morning. In my home, polishing shoes was a man's job and my father took pride in it. He got a feeling of satisfaction when he looked at the row of shoes ranging from the smallest to the largest, all gleaming back at him, with the look and smell of fresh polish.

Now, however, because of the onset of dementia, many gents cannot remember ever doing this polishing activity which was once part of their daily routine.

The Good News

Polishing shoes is very much a "muscle memory" activity. The steps involved are usually still there in the person's procedural memory, but have become buried and need to be resurrected. That is where we come in. Our job is to carefully devise activities which will help the person with dementia to re-activate that "muscle memory", so that once again, the person can polish his shoes and those of others and by doing so, feel useful again and feel that he is making a contribution to others.

Once again, it must be stated that making a contribution to others enhances a person's self-esteem. This is true of the human being at any age. Enhanced self-esteem always reduces anxiety and depression. A reduction of anxiety and depression results in more positive behaviour and less "responsive" behaviour and so a cycle of positivity begins.

Once again, if we can achieve all of this positive psychological health, simply by helping a person to remember how to polish shoes, we will have achieved something very significant indeed.

Motto
"Remind me how to do things for others."

POLISHING SHOES (Indirect Approach).

Preliminary Activity: Using a thick stick of chalk to colour shapes on a small blackboard.

Aim: To "jog" the person's "muscular memory" so as to re-activate the person's subconscious ability to perform the physical actions required for polishing shoes.

Motto: "Prime the pump".

Materials:
- A tray that sits neatly on the lap containing:
- A small hand-held blackboard.
- 2 sticks of very thick chalk.
- 2 sponge erasers.

Procedure:
- Approach the person in a quite but friends manner and sit beside him.
- Ask "would you help me to colour in these 2 squares", (drawn on the b/board).
- If "yes", hand the person one of the thick sticks of chalk.
- With your own thick stick of chalk, start colouring in one of the squares.
- When colouring in the square, use slow and deliberate movements, holding the chalk between your thumb and forefinger, as an indirect preparation for holding the shoe polish bottle in the Target Activity which is to come next.
- When both squares are coloured in, admire them for a moment with the gent.
- Now, hand the gent a sponge eraser and together, start rubbing out the chalk squares.
- Invite the person to repeat the activity if he wants to.
- When finished, thank the person and pack away the material.

Motto
"Invite me to do things for others."

POLISHING SHOES   (Direct Approach).

Target Activity: Polishing shoes for one's self and others.

Aim: To re-activate and fix into a routine the person's "procedural ability" to polish shoes.

Goal: To encourage the person to do things for others so as to help him to feel worthwhile again.

Materials:
- A trolley on castors containing:
- A sheet of newspaper.
- A pair of men's black shoes.
- Liquid shoe polish with a sponge applicator top x2.
- Hand wipes (non-allergenic).

Procedure:
- Approach the person in a friendly manner and greet him/her.
- Ask, "Could you help me to polish these shoes?"
- If "yes", lift one of the shoes off the trolley.
- Assuming you are right handed, place your left hand into the shoe to hold it steady. With your right hand, lift up the liquid polish (lid already off), and start to apply the polish to the shoe.
- After a minute or so, put down the shoe and polish and say "Would you like to help me?"
- If "yes", allow the person to place their left hand into the shoe. Now place the bottle of liquid polish (with the lid off) into their right hand or vice-versa.
- Allow the person time to register that they must rub the polish on the shoe.
- If the person does not do this, give assistance but back away as soon as they get the hang of it.
- Allow the person plenty of time to enjoy the activity.
- When the person is finished, thank him/her for their help.
- Ask if he/she would like to do the task again some other day.

EXTENSIONS TO THE EVERYDAY LIFE ACTIVITIES:

PRELIMINARY ACTIVITIES:
   (These activities may be offered, even to persons with severe dementia).

To strengthen the person's finger muscles and to promote dexterity of the hands, encourage the following Montessori Practical Life Activities.

- Opening and closing lids on jars.
- Opening and closing tops on bottles.
- Using tongs to transfer items from one bowl to another.
- Using tweezers to transfer items from one bowl to another.

(The following activities may be offered to persons with less severe dementia).

CARE OF ONE'S SELF:
- Trimming fingernails with a safety nail clippers.
- Shaving using a battery operated razor.
- Cleaning one's dentures.

CARE OF ONE'S ENVIRONMENT:
- Washing/drying dishes.
- Dusting furniture.
- Polishing brass/silver.
- Folding napkins.
- Packing away groceries in a food cabinet.
- Cleaning up small spills with a sponge.
- Washing a small table top with a sponge.
- Wiping a tray with a sponge.
- Wringing out wet sponges or face flannels.
- Hanging clothes on hangers.
- Putting clean clothes in drawers.

CARE OF OTHERS:
- Preparing a snack for a visitor by:
- Buttering bread,
- Slicing bananas,
- Putting biscuits on a plate.
- Arranging tea-cakes on a cake stand.

PART 3
SENSORY ACTIVITIES

Things To Ponder

Most people living with dementia are over 65 years of age. This means that for over 65 years they have smelled, tasted, touched, listened to and looked at, the world around them, developing their knowledge and understanding of their world in the process.

Now, because of this disability, their capacity to use their senses to experience and interpret the world them is often impeded.

Our job then, is to find ways to alleviate this problem.

The Good News

The Montessori Method, which is built on the original work of two French doctors, Itard and Sequin, is very much about "reaching the brain through the senses."

Dr. Maria Montessori, discovered through her painstaking experiments, that even the brains of children locked in a silent world of mental illness, could be reached by a carefully planned programme of sensory stimulation and training.

No matter what age we are, it is still possible to "reach our brains through our senses," and that is one of the chief aims of Montessori-Based Programmes for people living with Dementia.

In her original work, Dr. Montessori focused on each sense separately, using a very specific and scientific approach.

Here follows a simplified version of her approach that could be used with people living with dementia.

SIGHT	(Direct Approach step 1).
Preliminary Activity:	**Looking** at different colours, shapes and sizes.
Aim:	To "subliminally" motivate the person to notice things that **LOOK** the same.
Motto:	"Prime the pump."

Materials:
- "A book of things that **LOOK** the same".
- A tailor-made book on which the left and right hand pages contain pictures of identical items that are either the same colour, the same shape, or the same size. Eg:-

- 2 pictures of a large shoe, with size 12 written on them.
- 2 pictures of a large geometric figure.
- 2 pictures of a large pair of living room curtains.

Procedure:
- Approach the person in a friendly manner.
- Sit beside the person (to their dominant side).
- Greet the person and say something like "Could I show you this book?"
- If the person says "yes", open the book. The left hand page should have a coloured photo of an item and the right hand page should have an identical photo.
- Say "They **look** the same. don't they. They are the same size". Next, "They **look** the same, don't they. They are the same shape." Next, "They **look** the same, don't they. They are the same colour".
- Your aim is to revive the habit of noticing things that LOOK the same in the person's subconscious mind.
- Don't talk about extraneous matters, keep the focus on things that LOOK the same. For this reason, use very little speech, just point and say "same colour", "same shape", or "same size" as appropriate.
- When you reach the end of the book, ask the person if he/she wants to look through it again.
- Remember, repetition is the key to fixing things in the brain.
- When the activity is finished, thank the person for his/her co-operation.
- Ask the person if he/she would like to look at the book again some other day.

SIGHT	(Direct Approach step 2).
Target Activity:	Match things that **LOOK** the same.
Aim:	To re-activate the person's ability to match things that **LOOK** the same.
Goal:	To motivate the person to engage in meaningful activity, i.e. "work".
Activity:	Matching socks by colour.

Materials:
- A trolley on castors on which is placed:
- A wicker basket containing:
- 5 pairs of socks. (The socks should be in plain colours, not patterned and they should be identical in size and shape and should only differ in colour).
- Eg 1 blue pair, 1 red pair, 1 green pair, 1 brown pair and 1 yellow pair.

Procedure:
- Approach the person a friendly manner.
- Sit beside the person (to his/her dominant side).
- Greet the person and ask "Please, could you help me to match up these socks?"
- Empty the contents of the wicker basket onto the trolley.
- Say, something like "Oh dear, these socks are all mixed up".
- Slowly and deliberately, lift a red sock and say "Here's a red one, now I wonder where the matching red one is?"
- Again slowly and deliberately, reach your hand over and pick up the matching red sock.
- Place the two socks side by side on the trolley.
- Look at them closely as if to ascertain that they are the same colour.
- Indicate, with gesture of your hand that it is now the person's turn to match some socks.
- Allow the person plenty of time to get into the swing of the activity.
- When the person has matched one set, encourage him/her to match the next.
- When all the socks are matched up correctly, say something like, "Didn't we do a great job, they're all matched up now."
- Thank the person and put away the trolley.
- Extensions to this activity could be - matching "days of the week socks", which would also encourage reading skills, matching "stripy socks", matching "spotty socks" etc.

SOUND   (Direct Approach step 1).

Preliminary Activity: **Listening** to different sounds.

Aim: To "subliminally" motivate the person to notice things that **SOUND** the same.

Motto: "Prime the pump".

Materials:
- "A book of things that **SOUND** the same".
- A tailor-made book on which the left and right hand pages contain pouches in which are placed little boxes of items which produce an identical sound. Eg:-
- 2 boxes containing paper clips.
- 2 boxes containing marbles.
- 2 boxes containing erasers.
- 2 boxes containing lentils.
- 2 boxes containing beads.

Note: all the boxes should be sealed to prevent a choking hazard.

Procedure:
- Approach the person in a friendly way, introduce yourself and greet him/her.
- Sit beside the person and ask, "May I show you this book?"
- If "yes" open the book and lift out the box of p/clips from the left hand pouch.
- Hold the box of paper clips up to your left ear and shake it.
- Pass the box to the person and indicate that it is his/her turn to do this.
- Next, slowly lift out the box of paper clips from the right hand pouch.
- Hold the box up to your right ear and shake it.
- Pass the box to the person and indicate that it is his/her turn to do this.
- Now say, "they SOUND the same don't they."
- Now, slowly lift out the box containing marbles from the right hand pouch.
- Hold the box up to your right ear and shake it.
- Pass the box to the person and indicate that it is his/her turn to do this.
- Now say, "they SOUND the same don't they".
- Repeat this process in exactly the same way with the rest of the book.
- When you reach the end, thank the person for his/her co-operation.
- Now, maybe offer to have a cup of tea with the person and who knows, they might start a conversation about things that SOUND the same!

SOUND   (Direct Approach step 2).

Target Activity: Match things that **SOUND** the same.

Aim: To re-activate the person's ability to match things that **SOUND** the same.

Goal: To motivate the person to engage in meaningful activity, i.e "work".

Materials:
- A trolley on castors containing:
- A large box filled with a number of musical instruments all mixed up together, but including 2 maracas, 2 small drums with drum sticks, 2 small toy pianos, 2 small guitars and 2 tambourines.

Procedure:
- Approach the person in a friendly manner and greet him/her.
- Sit beside the person and introduce yourself.
- Ask, "May I show you this box of musical instruments?"
- If "yes", reach slowly into the box and let your fingers hit some notes on the piano.
- Lift out the piano.
- Next, reach into the box and let your fingers hit some notes on the second piano.
- Lift out the second piano.
- Say, "These pianos sound the same, don't they."
- Pass the two pianos to the person and allow him/her time to play a few notes on each one.
- Say again "They sound the same , don't they."
- Now invite the person to reach into the box and select a musical instrument.
- Invite the person to make a sound with the instrument,e.g beat the drum.
- Now invite the person to find another instrument that makes the same sound.
- Help the person to locate and make a sound on the second drum.
- Try to keep the emphasis on sound not sight.
- Say, "These drums **sound** the same, don't they.
- Allow the person plenty of time to register the point of the activity.
- Now, invite the person to reach into the box and select another instrument.
- Keep going until all 10 instruments have been matched up.
- Finally, thank the person for his/her co-operation.
- Maybe suggest a little "jam session" with the instruments!

TOUCH	(Direct Approach 1).
Preliminary Activity:	**Feeling** different textures.
Aim:	To "subliminally" motivate the person to notice textures that **FEEL** the same.
Motto:	"Prime the pump".

Materials:
- "A book of things that **FEEL** the same".
- A tailor-made book on which the left-hand and right-hand pages contain glued on swatches of identical fabrics.
- Eg.
- 2 identical swatches of velvet.
- 2 identical swatches of leather.
- 2 identical swatches of cotton.
- 2 identical swatches of silk.
- 2 identical swatches of lace.

Procedure:
- Approach the person in a friendly manner.
- Sit beside the person (to their dominant side).
- Greet the person and say something like, "Could I show you this lovely book?'
- If "yes", open the book. The left-hand page should have a swatch of fabric and the right hand page should have a swatch of identical fabric.
- Slowly and deliberately, feel the left hand swatch with your dominant hand.
- Say something like, "my, just feel this fabric, isn't it so soft and smooth".
- Then, reaching over to the right hand swatch do exactly the same.
- Say, "My, this one feels just the same, soft and smooth".
- Then allow the person to feel the left and right swatches just as you did.
- Now say, "They **feel** the same, don't they."
- Now, turn the page and repeat these steps with the next set of swatches.
- Say, "They feel the same, don't they".
- Now invite the person to feel the next pair of swatches and the next until he/she has felt all of them.
- Always remember to say, "They feel the same, don't they".
- When finished, thank the person and ask if he/she enjoyed the activity and if he/she would like to do the activity again on another day.
- Lastly, put the material away.

TOUCH	(Direct Approach step 2).
Target Activity:	Match things that **FEEL** the same.
Aim:	To re-activate the person's ability to match things that **FEEL** the same.
Goal:	To motivate the person to engage in meaningful activity, i.e. "work".
Activity:	Matching gloves by texture.

Materials:
- A trolley on castors on which is placed a basket containing:
- 5 pairs of gloves and 5 clothes pegs.
- All the gloves should be the same colour, the same size and the same shape. They should only differ in texture. Eg.1 pair of leather gloves, 1 pair of woollen gloves, 1 pair of velvet gloves,1 pair of rubber gloves, 1 pair of garden gloves.

Procedure:
- Approach the person in a friendly manner and greet him/her.
- Sit beside the person to their dominant side and introduce yourself.
- Ask, "Please, could you help me to match up these gloves?"
- Empty the contents of the wicker basket onto the trolley.
- Say something like, "Oh, my goodness, the gloves are all mixed up".
- Slowly and deliberately, lift up a leather glove, feel its texture carefully and say "This is a leather glove, now I wonder, where the matching leather glove is?"
- Slowly and deliberately reach your hand over the pile of mixed up gloves and pick up the matching leather glove. Place the two side by side on the trolley.
- Feel them slowly and carefully to ascertain that they are the same texture.
- Now, indicate with your hand that it is the person's turn to match some gloves.
- Allow the person plenty of time to select a glove. When he/she has selected a glove, encourage him/her to thoroughly feel the glove to identify its texture.
- Now, encourage the person to look for the matching glove.
- Avoid talking as it may confuse the person. Try to keep the focus on feeling the textures of the gloves and matching up gloves with identical textures.
- Encourage the person to keep matching up the gloves.
- When all the gloves have been matched, hopefully by the person him/herself, say something like, "Well didn't we do a great job. We matched all the gloves".
- Ask the person if he/she enjoyed the activity. If the answer is "yes", ask if he/she would like to do it again some other day. Remember to thank the person.

TASTE	(Direct Approach step 1).
Preliminary Activity:	**Tasting** different flavours.
Aim:	To "subliminally" motivate the person to notice things that **TASTE** the same.
Motto:	"Prime the pump".

Materials:
- "A book of things that **TASTE** the same".
- A tailor-made book on which the left and right hand pages contain little pouches in which you may place little bags of items which have an identical flavour. Eg.
- 2 x Small Bars of chocolate.
- 2 x Shortbread biscuits.
- 2 x Pieces of Fudge.
- 2 x Strawberry Nutrigrain Bars.
- 2 x Slices of Fruitcake.

Procedure:
- Approach the person in a friendly manner and greet him/her.
- Sit beside the person and ask "May I show you this book?'
- If "yes", open the book and carefully lift out the bar of chocolate from the left hand pouch.
- Break a piece off the bar and taste it.
- Pass a piece to the person and indicate that it is his/her turn to taste it.
- Next, carefully lift out the bar of chocolate from the right hand pouch.
- Break a piece off the bar and taste it.
- Pass a piece to the person and indicate that it is his/her turn to taste it.
- Now say, "They **taste** the same, don't they".
- Now, slowly lift out a shortbread biscuit from the right hand pouch.
- Break a piece off and taste it.
- Pass a piece to the person and indicate that it is his/her turn to taste it.
- Now say, "They taste the same, don't they".
- Repeat this process in exactly the same way with the rest of the book.
- When you reach the end, thank the person for his/her co-operation.
- Maybe suggest that you have a cup of tea or coffee together and enjoy the rest of that chocolate!

TASTE   (Direct Approach 2).

Target Activity: Match things that **TASTE** the same.

Aim: To re-activate the person's ability to match things that **TASTE** the same.

Goal: To motivate the person to engage in meaningful activity, i.e., "work".

Materials:
- 10 cupcakes on a large plate, comprising of:
- 2 with coffee icing, 2 with lemon icing, 2 with strawberry icing, 2 with mint icing and 2 with blueberry icing.
- 1 square plate.
- 1 knife.
- 10 little stick-on labels with the icing name on them.

Procedure:
- Approach the person in a friendly manner and greet him/her.
- Sit beside the person and introduce yourself.
- Ask, "Would you like to taste these lovely cakes with me?"
- If "yes", reach over to the plate, select a cake, cut it into 3 pieces and give the first piece to the person to taste, the second to yourself to taste and place the third on the square plate.
- Say, "This tastes like lemon". (or whatever).
- Now, take the label that says "lemon" and put it beside the piece on the plate.
- Now, reach over to the large plate and select another cake, cut it into 3 pieces and give the first piece to the person to taste while you taste the second piece and place the third piece on the square plate.
- Say, "This tastes like coffee". (or whatever).
- Now, take the label that says "coffee" and put it beside the piece on the plate.
- Continue like this until all the cakes have been tasted and labelled.
- Now, match up the labels, i.e. put the piece of lemon cake alongside the other piece of lemon cake, the piece of coffee cake along side the other piece of coffee cake etc.
- Say, • "Those two are lemon cakes, those two are coffee cakes, those two are mint cakes, those two are strawberry cakes and those two are blueberry cakes".
- Finally, thank the person for his/her co-operation, and maybe invite a third person to come and have tea and cake with you both!

SMELL   (Direct Approach step 1).

Preliminary Activity: **Smelling** different aromas.

Aim: To "subliminally" motivate the person
                                               to notice things that **SMELL** the same.

Motto: "Prime the pump".

Materials:
- "A book of things that **SMELL** the same".
- A tailor-made book in which the left and right hand paged contain little pouches in which may be placed identical items that have an identical smell.
- 2 bags containing dried lavender.
- 2 bags containing dried herbs.
- 2 bags containing pieces of pinewood.
- 2 bags containing cinnamon sticks.
- 2 bags containing carbolic soap.

Procedure:
- Approach the person in a friendly manner and greet him/her.
- Sit beside the person and ask, "May I show you this book?"
- If "yes", open the book and slowly lift out the bag of dried lavender from the left hand pouch.
- Open the bag and smell the lavender.
- Pass the bag of lavender to the person and indicate that it is his/her turn to smell it.
- Next, slowly lift out the bag of lavender from the right hand pouch.
- Open the bag and smell the lavender.
- Now, pass the second bag of lavender to the person and indicate that it is his/her turn to smell it.
- Now say, "They **smell** the same, don't they".
- Now, slowly lift out the bag of dried herbs from the left hand pouch.
- Open the bag and smell the herbs.
- Pass the bag of herbs to the person and indicate that he/she should smell it.
- Next, slowly lift out the bag of herbs from the right hand pouch.
- Open the bag and smell the herbs.
- Repeat the process as outlined above, with the herbs and the rest of the book.
- When you reach the end, thank the person for his/her co-operation.
- Maybe suggest that you go out to the garden together and smell some fresh plants and flowers.

SMELL: (Direct Approach step 2).

Target Activity: Match things that **SMELL** the same.

Aim: To re-activate the person's ability to match things that **SMELL** the same.

Goal: To motivate the person to engage in meaningful activity, i.e "work".

Materials:
- 1 basket containing:
2 x Roses.
2 x Wallflowers.
2 x Honeysuckle.
2 x Lavender
2 x Lilies

Procedure:
- Approach the person in a friendly manner and greet him/her.
- Sit beside the person and introduce yourself.
- Ask, "Would you like to smell these lovely flowers with me?"
- If "yes", reach over to the basket of flowers and take out a rose.
- Lift the rose close to you nose and smell it.
- Say, "This smells like a rose".
- Pass the rose to the person and indicate that it is his/her turn to smell it.
- Allow the person enough time to smell it., then say again, "It smells like a rose".
- Now, take a label that says "rose" and lie the rose on the trolley beside the label.
- Now reach over to the basket and take out a clipping of honeysuckle.
- Lift the honeysuckle close to your nose and smell it.
- Say, "This smells like honeysuckle".
- Pass the clipping of honeysuckle to the person and indicate that it is his/her turn to smell it.
- Allow the person enough time to smell it, then say, "It smells like honeysuckle".
- Take a label that says "honeysuckle" and lie it and the clipping on the trolley.
- Continue in this manner until all the flowers have been smelled and labelled.
- Now start to match up the flowers with the labels.
- Say to the person, "We'll put a rose beside a rose because they smell the same, and a wallflower beside a wallflower because they smell the same," etc.
- When all the flowers have been matched up according to smell, thank the person for his/her co-operation.

EXTENSIONS TO THE SENSORIAL ACTIVITIES

SIGHT: To help to preserve the person's visual sense, encourage activities using the following Montessori materials:

- The knobbed cylinders.
- The Pink Tower.
- The knob-less cylinders.
- The Geometric Cabinet.
- The Colour Tablets.

SOUND: To help to preserve the person's auditory sense, encourage activities using the following Montessori materials:

- The Sound Cylinders.

TOUCH: To help to preserve the person's tactile sense, encourage activities using the following Montessori materials.

- The Touch Boards.
- The Tactile Tablets.
- The Fabric Boxes.

TASTE: To help to preserve the person's gustatory sense, encourage activities using the following Montessori materials.

- The Tasting Cups.

SMELL: To help to preserve the person's olfactory sense, encourage activities using the following Montessori materials.

- The Smell Jars.

NOTE: One should be shown how to use these materials by a trained Montessori practitioner.

PART 4
LANGUAGE ACTIVITIES

TALKING

Things To Ponder

One of the saddest facts about dementia is that it frequently robs the person of the ability to talk normally. The onset of dementia can cause the person to develop a host of language problems. These often include, forgetting words, mixing up words or just not speaking words any more.

There are many reasons why people living with dementia stop talking. Some are entirely medical and there are all sorts of complex names for these conditions.

But, some of the reasons why people living with dementia, stop talking are not so complex, in fact, they are very simple. The person may feel sad, depressed, lonely, lost, frightened or just not themselves anymore.

The Good News

Even when someone living with dementia has developed language problems, it is never too late to introduce language activities which may help to support the language skills the person still has and even halt further decline.

Some experts say that we cannot stop the inevitable deterioration of language skills in a progressive disease like dementia. Our response is, we have nothing to lose by trying to halt that progression, and what if we do halt it even by a small degree, isn't that still worthwhile?

With these things in mind, let's see how we might go about helping a person living with dementia to re-activate the ability to talk.

The approach has two stages. Firstly, our job is to **subliminally** "prime the pump" of procedural memory and secondly to **consciously**, re-activate the "habit" of talking in the person living with dementia, once again.

Motto
"Help me to remember how to talk."

TALKING   (Indirect Approach).

Preliminary Activities: Listening while someone speaks. Watching someone's mouth as they speak. Mimicking speech silently.

Aim: To "jog" the "procedural" memory" so as to re-activate the person's "subconscious ability" to pronounce words and put sentences together, without having to consciously think about it.

Motto: "Prime the pump."

Materials:
- One kind-hearted individual willing to sit with a person living with dementia and talk to him/her for about 15 minutes a day, even if the person does not initially respond, or even look as if he/she is listening to what's being said.
- A smile.
- A willingness to hold the person's hand, if needed.

Procedure:
- Approach the person in a friendly manner and greet him/her.
- Sit beside the person and introduce yourself.
- Say, "Would it be ok for me to sit and chat to you for a while?"
- Talk about the weather, the nice flowers on the table (that you have brought, perhaps), the nice cup of tea that you are both drinking etc.
- The importance is not so much in what you talk about, but in the fact that you are talking, thus priming the pump of the person's procedural memory.
- Remember to look at the person as you speak so that he/she can watch your mouth moving. (This is how we all initially pick up language as infants, and it is also an effective way to re-activate speech in someone who has lost their speech following emotional trauma.
- After about 15 minutes, smile, say, "It's been a pleasure talking to you, may I come again sometime to chat with you?"

Motto
"Encourage me to talk everyday."

TALKING	(Direct Approach).
Target Activity:	Using speech to communicate.
Aim:	To re-activate and "fix" into a routine the person's "subconscious ability" to communicate with others through speech.
Goal:	To motivate the person to "talk".

Materials:
- Another kind-hearted person willing to sit with a person living with dementia and talk to him/her for about 15 minutes a day.
- An activity that supports a 2-way conversation, (in this example, the activity is looking at a cookery book with large coloured pictures of delicious foods).
- A friendly smile.

Procedure:
- Approach the person in a friendly manner and greet him/her.
- Sit beside the person and introduce yourself.
- Say, "Could I show you what I have here?"
- If "yes", take out the activity. (In this scenario, it is a cookery book).
- Open a page which has a large photo of a delicious cake on it.
- Say, with a smile on your face, "Oh my, that looks delicious doesn't it?"
- Allow a few moments for the person to respond. If he/she doesn't respond, don't be disheartened, just continue.
- Open another page which has a large photo of a delicious meal on it.
- Say, (laughing), "Oh, that's making me hungry! Is it making you hungry too?"
- Wait for an answer. If none comes, just continue happily.
- Open another page and continue as before.
- Even if there is no response keep turning the pages and talking enthusiastically.
- If you do this regularly, there is a very strong likelihood that the person will begin to talk again. Even people who haven't talked for years have been known to begin talking again following this process. Never give up.
- At the end of the session, say, "It's been a pleasure talking to you", (use the person's name), "I hope we can have a chat together again sometime soon".

WRITING

Things To Ponder

Writing is an extraordinary skill. It enables us to transmit the very thoughts in our heads, through squiggles on paper, to others. This is not something we should take for granted. It is an extraordinary invention and an indescribably valuable skill.

Most people, in the developed world will have learned to write as a child. This means that he/she has had this skill for about 60 or 70 years. Some people will have made more use of this skill than others, but the skill is there nevertheless.

Now the other extraordinary thing about the skill of writing is that the ability to write is stored in our procedural or "muscle memory". How do we know this? Well, there have been some amazing documented cases of people who, having suffered a blow to the head, subsequently developed amnesia. They couldn't remember who they were. Yet, and this is the amazing thing, if given paper and a pen, they could write their signature.

So, even though they couldn't remember their name, (due to semantic memory damage), they could still write their signature. This means that the ability to write is not affected by damage to the semantic memory, because the ability to write is clearly stored in "procedural memory".

The Good News

This is clearly good news for the person living with dementia. What this means is that the skill of writing may be re-activated in the person living with dementia, if we "prime the pump" of procedural memory.

Our job therefore, is two-fold. Firstly, we need to "subliminally "prime the pump" of procedural memory and secondly, to consciously re-activate the "habit" of writing in the person with dementia.

Let's have a look at how we might go about this.

Motto
"Remind me how to make letter shapes."

WRITING	(Indirect Approach).
Preliminary Activity:	Making shapes in sand with the forefinger of the dominant hand.
Aim:	To "jog" the person's "muscular memory" so as to re-activate the person's "subconscious ability" to perform the physical actions involved in writing.
Motto:	"Prime the pump"

Materials:
- A trolley on castors containing:
- A sand tray filled with a layer of sand.
- A wooden dowel pointed like a pencil and a wooden lat to erase.

Procedure:
- Approach the person in a quite but friendly manner.
- Sit beside the person to their dominant side.
- Ask "Can I show you this?"
- If "yes", place the trolley in front of yourself and the person.
- Lift up the wooden dowel.
- Slowly and deliberately, begin to make a letter shape in the sand.
- Now wipe it out with the wooden eraser and very slowly and deliberately make another letter. (Initially, never write more than one letter at a time).
- After you have had about three turns, hand the dowel to the person and indicate with a gesture that he/she may have a turn.
- Allow the person plenty of time to write a letter shape.
- Show the person how to use the wooden lat to erase each letter.
- If the person shows interest, invite him/her to write their name in the sand.
- If they show a strong interest in this activity invite them to write the names of their children or grandchildren in the sand.
- Help the person to think up words to write.
- When the person has had enough, thank him/her and and ask if he/she enjoyed the game. Finally, put the materials away till next time.

Motto
"Encourage me to write words and phrases."

WRITING (Direct Approach).

Target Activity: Writing with a pen/pencil.

Aim: To re-activate and "fix" into a routine the person's "subconscious ability" to write.

Materials:
- A trolley on castors.
- An A5 size drawing pad. (blank, no lines).
- Some blank greeting cards.
- 2 x Pens /pencils.
- (If the person has arthritis a thick pencil with a finger grip would be helpful).

Procedure:
- Approach the person in a friendly manner.
- Sit beside the person to their dominant side.
- Ask, "Would you like to see what I've got here?"
- If "yes", place the trolley in front of yourself and the person.
- Say, "I've got some paper and pens here and some lovely cards".
- Show the writing materials to the person.
- Allow the person plenty of time to register what the materials are for.
- Say, "I think I'll write a card to my friend."
- Slowly and deliberately, pick up a pen or pencil and very deliberately start writing, "Dear Mary, I hope you are well".
- Speak the words aloud as you write.
- Now, stop and ask the person, "Would you like to write a card?"
- If "yes", pass a pencil to the person.
- Allow the person plenty of time to start the process.
- Don't talk if possible, as talk will distract the person, however if the person is chatty, be prepared to join in, possibly helping with ideas, (or spellings).
- When the person appears to be finished, offer to post the card.
- Finally, thank the person and leave him/her with some writing materials in the hope that this activity will have motivated the person to start writing again.

READING

Things To Ponder

Most persons, in the developed world, living with dementia, would have learned to read when he/she was a child. This means that they have been "reading" anything from road signs, to shop notices, to newspapers, to magazines, to books, for about 60 or 70 years. That's a long time.

During this time, reading would have become a habit, something they unconsciously did like the way we rub our eyes when we're tired or stretch our arms when we yawn.

We never consciously think about these actions, we just do them from habit. In the same way, we unconsciously read all the time.

As we sit in the kitchen having breakfast, we unconsciously read the back of the cereal packet, we unconsciously read the side of the milk carton, we unconsciously read the label on the bananas and the sticker on the apples in the fruit bowl. In fact, we read, read, read. all day long and we are not consciously aware of it.

The Good News

Now, the good news is, since reading is a habit, long ingrained into most of us, it can be re-activated, even in people who are aged and living with dementia. We just have to "prime the pump".

Our job, once again, is two-fold. Firstly, we need to "subliminally" "prime the pump" of procedural memory and secondly, to re-activate the habit of reading in persons living with dementia.

Let's see how we might go about doing this.

Motto
"Remind me that I can read."

READING	(Indirect Approach).

Preliminary Activity: Hanging up notices.

Aim: To "jog" the person's "muscular memory" so as to re-activate the person's "subconscious ability" to read.

Motto: "Prime the pump."

Materials:
- 10 laminated signs e.g. toilet, kitchen, cooker, fridge, toaster, kettle, cups and plates, knives, forks, spoons.
- Some sellotape.

Procedure:
- Approach the person in a friendly manner and greet him/her.
- Sit beside the person to their dominant side.
- Ask, "Could you help me to hang up these signs?"
- If "yes", ask the person, who may be in a wheel-chair, to hold the sellotape .
- Ask the person to walk with you or allow you to wheel him/her over to the position where you are intending to hang the first laminated sign.
- Say, "this sign says "TOILET", this will help people to know where the toilet is
- Hang up the sign, then say, now we need to hang up another sign.
- Select another sign and say, "this sign says, "KITCHEN", this will help people to know where the kitchen is.
- Hang up the sign, then say, now we need to hang up another sign.
- Invite the person to select another sign to hang up.
- Now ask, "Where should we put this?"
- Allow the person time to figure out the answer. Only prompt if necessary.
- Continue until all the signs are in position.
- If the person appears to be enjoying the activity ask, "What other signs do you think we should put up?"
- If the person makes suggestions, get some paper and a marker and make some more signs. Then, hang them up together.
- Finally, thank the person for his/her co-operation.

Motto
"Get me back into the habit of reading."

READING	(Direct Approach).
Target Activity:	Reading books, newspapers, magazines.
Aim:	To re-activate the "habit" of reading.
Goal:	To motivate the person to read again .

Materials:
- A selection of attractive looking books with large print, specially selected to relate to the person's former interests.
- A reading companion, (i.e a kind-hearted person with 15 - 20 minutes to spare, willing to sit beside the person with dementia and read with them or to them.

Procedure:
- Approach the person in a friendly manner and greet him/her.
- Sit beside the person to their dominant side.
- Ask, "Could I show you some books?"
- If "yes", select a book that you think might interest the person and read the title out loud. Eg. "Growing up in Ireland in the 1930's".
- Say, "That sounds interesting, shall I read a bit of it to you?"
- If "yes", open the book and slowly and distinctly, read a page or two.
- Now, say "Would you read this page while I"..... (look for my reading glasses/ fasten my lace/drink my tea/take off my coat, etc. i.e. make some excuse.)
- Encourage the person to read a page or two, filling in words for him/her, if necessary.
- Do everything you can to help the person to feel comfortable about reading aloud. This is best done by showing that you are very interested in the content he/she is reading out to you. Say things like, "My, that's very interesting, I never knew that" etc.
- If the person hands the book back to you, continue the reading yourself for as long as the person seems interested.
- When finished, thank the person saying , "I really enjoyed reading with you today, could we do it again sometime?"
- Lastly, offer to have a cup of tea and a chat with the person.
- Be alert, you never know the book may have stimulated conversation.

EXTENSIONS TO THE LANGUAGE ACTIVITIES

The following activities may be offered to persons who are living with a mild/moderate, i.e not a severe, level of dementia.

TALKING: To help to preserve the person's ability to talk and communicate using language, encourage the following Montessori activities:

- The I-Spy Game.
- Classification Cards (using concrete objects).
- Classification Cards (using pictures of everyday objects along with Control Cards which help to categorise the pictures into classes such as, Kitchen utensils and appliances, Sitting room furniture, Bathroom essentials, Bedroom furniture, Gardening tools, etc.
- These could be presented as intergenerational games to play with children/grandchildren).

WRITING: To help to preserve the person's writing skills, encourage tasks/activities using the following Montessori materials:

- The Insets for Design (Metal Insets).
- The Moveable Alphabet.
- The Sandpaper Letters
- Small Blackboards and chalk.

READING: To help to preserve the person's reading skills, encourage tasks/activities using the following Montessori materials:

- Object Boxes and Cards.
- Action Cards.
- Large Print Books.

NOTE: One should be shown how to use these materials by a trained Montessori practitioner.

PART 5
MATHEMATICAL ACTIVITIES

Things to Ponder

One of the problems encountered by people living with dementia is that people around them begin to assume that because they have impaired memory, they have lost all intelligence. This is just not so, but because of this widespread perception, we have a tendency not to offer anything intelligent to persons with dementia. This is a great mistake. Dr. Maria Montessori always pointed out that the human being is naturally mathematical. We are naturally predisposed to sort, match, compare, contrast and calculate every thing we see and touch around us. We do it all the time unconsciously.

While it is undeniable that at certain stages in dementia the person's cognitive skills can be hugely damaged, this should not dissuade us from offering "mathematical" type activities to person's with dementia so that whatever skills have been "spared" may be strengthened and put to good use.

The Good News

Experience has shown us that even people in late stage dementia can still perform and enjoy "mathematical" types of activities that involve sorting, matching, contrasting, comparing and even calculating. The key is to find the person's area of interest and to build the activity around that area.

For example, a lady who was primarily a homemaker will usually enjoy sorting clothes into categories because she will have had years of experience of doing this for her family.

Similarly, a gent who enjoyed fishing as a hobby will usually enjoy sorting out fishing tackle. Alternatively, a gent who enjoyed DIY will usually enjoy sorting out nuts, bolts, screws and tools.

Once we find out what the person's interests were, the possibilities for creating activities are endless.

With this in mind, let's look at how we might present "mathematical" types of activities to people living with dementia.

Motto
"Help me to use it, so I don't lose it."

SORTING.	Sorting according to size, shape, colour, texture, weight, length, height, etc.
Activity: (for Ladies).	Sorting buttons into categories.
Aim:	To protect the person's remaining cognitive strengths from decline and to try to build on them.
Goal:	To motivate the person to engage in meaningful activity, i.e. "work".

Materials:
- A wicker basket full of large and small buttons., (not medium at this point).
- 2 bowls marked "large" and "small".

Procedure:
- Approach the person in a friendly manner and greet her.
- Ask, "Could you help me to sort out all these buttons?"
- Slowly and deliberately, reach into the basket and take out a large button.
- Carefully and without any speech, place the button in the bowl marked "large".
- Now, slowly and deliberately, reach into the basket and take out a small button.
- Carefully and without any speech, place the button in the bowl marked "small".
- Repeat.
- Next, indicate to the person, using a hand gesture, that it is her turn to sort the buttons.
- Allow the person plenty of time to register what you are indicating.
- When the person selects a button, give her time to place the button in the correct bowl.
- If the person is hesitant about which bowl to put the button in, indicate the correct bowl by pointing, try not to talk as this may confuse the person.
- When the person has sorted the buttons, say "wow, you did a great job".
- Do not correct the person, even if some of the buttons are in the wrong bowls.
- Remember the goal of the activity is to motivate the person to do an activity.
- When the person is clearly finished, thank her for her help.

Motto
"Help me to use it ,so I don't lose it."

SORTING.	Sorting according to size, shape, colour, texture, weight, length, height, etc.
Activity: (for Gents).	Sorting nuts and bolts into categories.
Aim:	To protect the person's remaining cognitive strengths from decline and to try to build on them.
Goal:	To motivate the person to engage in meaningful activity, i.e. "work".

Materials:
- A box full of large and small nuts and bolts, (not medium at this point).
- 2 boxes marked "large" and "small".

Procedure:
- Approach the person in a friendly manner and greet him.
- Ask, "Would you help me to sort out these nuts and bolts?"
- Slowly and deliberately reach into the box of nuts and bolts and take out a large nut and bolt.
- Carefully and without any speech, place it into the box marked "large".
- Now, slowly and deliberately, reach into the box of nuts and bolts and take out a small nut and bolt.
- Carefully and without any speech, place the nut and bolt into the box marked "small".
- Repeat.
- Next, indicate to the person using a hand gesture that it is his turn to sort the nuts and bolts.
- Allow the person plenty of time to register what you are indicating.
- When the person selects a nut and bolt, give him time to place it in the correct box. Try not to interfere, even if he is slow in doing it.
- If the person is very hesitant about which box to put the nut and bolt into, indicate the correct box by pointing with your forefinger, but try not to talk.
- When the person has sorted all the nuts and bolts, say, "You did a great job."
- Do not correct the person even if some of the nuts and bolts are in the wrong boxes. Remember, the goal of the activity is to motivate the person to "work", i.e. engage in meaningful activity.
- When the person is clearly finished, thank him for his help.

Motto
"Help me to use it, so I don't lose it."

CONTRASTING.	According to temperature weight, height, etc.
Activity: (for Ladies).	Contrasting according to Weight.
Aim:	To protect the person's remaining cognitive strengths from decline and to try to build on them.
Goal:	To motivate the person to engage in meaningful activity, i.e. "work".

Materials:
- 1 box containing the following:
- 10 silver plaited tea-spoons.
- 10 silver coloured plastic spoons.
- 2 cutlery trays, one marked silver plaited spoons and the other marked plastic spoons.

Procedure:
- Approach the lady in a friendly manner and greet her.
- Sit beside the lady to her dominant side and introduce yourself.
- Ask, "Could you help me to sort out these spoons?"
- If "yes", slowly reach into the box and take out a silver plaited tea-spoon.
- Let it rest across the palm of your hand and say, "My this is "heavy".
- Now, slowly, place the silver plaited spoon in the cutlery tray marked "silver plaited spoons".
- Now, slowly reach into the box and take out a silver coloured plastic spoon.
- Let it rest across the palm of your hand and say, "My, this "light".
- Now, slowly place the the silver coloured plastic spoon in the cutlery tray marked "plastic spoons".
- Now, indicate with a hand gesture that it is the person's turn to do the activity.
- Allow the person plenty of time to reach for a spoon and put it in a box.
- Try to avoid interfering even if the person is taking a long time to do anything.
- If the person appears to be really confused about what to do, indicate with your finger which box she should be reaching towards.
- When all the spoon have been sorted, smile and thank the lady.

Motto
"Help me to use it, so I don't lose it."

CONTRASTING.	According to temperature, weight, height, etc.
Activity: (for Gents).	Contrasting according to Weight.
Aim:	To protect the person's remaining cognitive strengths from decline and to try to build on them.
Goal:	To motivate the person to engage in meaningful activity, i.e. "work".

Materials:
- 1 wooden box containing the following:
- 10 white golf balls.
- 10 white ping pong balls.
- 2 smaller wooden boxes marked LIGHT and HEAVY.

Procedure:
- Approach the person in a friendly manner and greet him.
- Sit beside the gent to his dominant side and introduce yourself.
- Ask, "Could you help me to sort out these balls?"
- If "yes", slowly reach into the wooden box and take out a golf ball.
- Let it rest in the palm of your hand say, "My, that's "heavy".
- Now, slowly place the ping pong ball in the box marked "heavy".
- Now, slowly reach into the wooden box and take out a ping pong ball.
- Let it rest in the palm of your hand and say, "My, that's "light".
- Now, slowly place the ping pong ball in the box marked "light".
- Now, indicate, with a gesture of your hand that it is now the person's turn to have a go at the activity.
- Allow the person plenty of time to reach for a ball and decide which box it should go into.
- Try to avoid interfering even if the person is slow about doing the activity.
- If the person appears confused about where to put a ball that he has chosen, give help by pointing with your forefinger to the correct box. Try not to talk if possible as talking will probably confuse the person.
- When all the balls have been sorted, smile and thank the person.

Motto
"Help me to use it, so I don't lose it."

MATCHING.	Quantity to Numeral.
Activity: (for Ladies).	Matching quantities of sweets with numeral cards.
Aim:	To protect the person's remaining cognitive strengths from decline and to try to build on them.
Goal:	To motivate the person to engage in meaningful activity, i.e. "work".

Materials:
- A trolley on castors.
- 1 wicker basket.
- 10 small bowls.
- 55 sweets wrapped in identical coloured wrappers.
- Numeral cards 1 to 10.

Procedure:
- Approach the person in a friendly manner and greet her.
- Sit beside the lady to her dominant side and introduce yourself.
- Ask, "Could you help me to count out these sweets?"
- If "yes", lay out the numeral cards on the trolley, in sequence from 1 to 10.
- Now, slowly reach into the basket and take out 1 sweet and say clearly and distinctly, "ONE".
- Place the sweet under the numeral 1.
- Now, slowly reach into the basket and take out 2 sweets and say, clearly and distinctly, "TWO".
- Place the 2 sweets under the numeral 2.
- Now, indicate with a gesture of your hand that it is the lady's turn to try the activity.
- Allow the lady plenty of time to select some sweets from the basket.
- If the lady looks to you for clarification on how many sweets she should take, say, "THREE", and hold up 3 fingers.
- Allow the lady enough time to lay out the three sweets under the numeral 3.
- Now, indicate to the lady to reach for more sweets to match to numeral card 4.
- When all the numerals have been matched with sweets, say "wow, that's great".
- When the activity is clearly finished, remember to thank the lady for her help.

Motto
"Help me to use it, so I don't lose it."

MATCHING.

Quantity to Numeral.

Activity: (for Gents).

Matching quantities of poker chips with numeral cards.

Aim:

To protect the person's remaining cognitive strengths from decline and to try to build on them.

Goal:

To motivate the person to engage in meaningful activity, i.e "work".

Materials:
- 1 trolley on castors.
- 1 wooden box.
- 10 small boxes.
- 55 poker chips.
- Numeral cards 1 to 10.

Procedure:
- Approach the person in a friendly manner and greet him.
- Sit beside the gent to his dominant side and introduce yourself.
- Ask, "Could you help me to count out these poker chips?"
- If "yes", lay out the numeral cards on the trolley in sequence from 1 to 10.
- Now slowly reach into the box and take out one poker chip and say clearly and distinctly, "ONE".
- Place the poker chip under the numeral 1.
- Now, slowly reach into the box and take out 2 poker chips and say, clearly and distinctly, "TWO".
- Place the 2 poker chips under the numeral 2.
- Now, indicate with a gesture of your hand that it is the gent's turn to try the activity.
- Allow the gent plenty of time to select some poker chips from the box.
- If the gent looks towards you for clarification on how many poker chips he should select, say, "THREE", and hold up 3 fingers.
- Allow the gent enough time to lay out the 3 poker chips under the numeral 3.
- Now, indicate to the gent to reach for more poker chips to match the 4 card.
- When all the numerals have been matched with poker chips, say, "Great job".
- When the gent is clearly finished doing the activity, remember to thank him.

EXTENSIONS TO THE MATHEMATICAL ACTIVITIES.

The following activities may be offered to persons who are living with a mild/moderate, level of dementia.

Numeracy: To help to preserve the person's numerical skills, encourage activities using the following mathematical materials:

- The Spindle Boxes.
- The Number Cards and Counters.
- The Teen Boards.
- The Tens Boards.
- The 100 square.
- Selections of the Golden Bead Material.
- Number cards 1 to 9000.

Cognition: To help to preserve the person's cognitive strengths, encourage activities using the following materials.

- The Binomial Cube.
- The Trinomial Cube.
- The Fraction Circles.
- The Division Board.
- The Multiplication Board.

Uniqueness of the Montessori maths. materials for people with dementia.
The unique advantage of the Montessori mathematical materials for people living with dementia is their "concreteness". The materials are tangible and concrete. They do not require the person to imagine abstractions. Remember, when someone is living with dementia, "out of sight" often means "out of mind". Therefore the Montessori mathematical materials are unique in that they keep the mathematical problem "literally" in front of the person, in a concrete form.

NOTE: One should be shown how to use these materials by a trained Montessori practitioner.

PART 6
CULTURAL ACTIVITIES

Things To Ponder.

One of the problems encountered by persons living with dementia is that the disability can quench their motivation and interest in everything. Hobbies, interests, passions, can all be cast aside as the person becomes enveloped in a sad, lonely prison of apathy.

Some of the reasons for this apathy are medical and have a lot to do with levels of hormones especially dopamine in the brain. But some of the reasons for this apathy are less complex and have more to do with normal human emotions like, anger and frustration at the loss of physical dexterity, loneliness as family and friends seem to visit less, sadness as one realises that old age is catching up on one and cannot be prevented and annoyance that our memory is not what it used to be.

Our job therefore is to find ways of helping people living with dementia to overcome some of these problems and break out of these sad, prisons of apathy.

The Good News.

Our experience tells us that it is never too late to awaken a person and revive an interest in something. Most persons living with dementia have spent over 50 years acquiring what we call "culture".

"Culture", is an umbrella term. It embraces things like our history, our heritage, our traditions, our families, our pastimes, our hobbies, our passions, our music, song and dance and our spiritual beliefs.

There is a huge store-house of "culture" locked inside every person living with dementia. Our job then, is to open the door to that store-house and let some of that 50 or 60 years of acquired culture come to the surface.

With this in mind, let's have a look at how we might present activities to persons living with dementia which may unlock the door to their specifically acquired culture and help them to remember, who they are, where they came from, what they used to enjoy doing, what music they liked to listen to, what kept them active, what they lived through, what they identified with, what they celebrated and what gave them meaning. All of this, is what we call "culture."

Motto
"Help me to remember who I am."

FAMILY:	(Who I Am).

Aim: To help the person to "remember" who he/she is and what family he/she belongs to.

Activity: Flicking through a family photo album.

Materials:
- A trolley on castors on which is placed:
- A photo album, put together by someone who is close to the person living with dementia. (This is a crucial step in the process. Many people have family members they would rather forget, those who have upset or even abused them. There should be no trace of these people in the family album).
- Labels under the photos stating the name of the person in the photo and their relation to the person with dementia.

Procedure:
- Approach the person in a friendly manner greet him/her.
- Sit beside the person to his/her dominant side and introduce yourself.
- Ask, "Would you like to look at these photos?"
- If "yes", open the album at the first page and comment on the photos.
- Do NOT ask the person questions like "who's that?" or "what's her name?" or make comments like "surely, you must remember him, you were married to him for 40 years!" Questions and comments like this only make the person feel demoralised if he/she cannot remember the names of the persons in the photos or even who the persons in the photos are. This is the advantage of having names and identities already written underneath each photo so that you can say things like, "Oh, this is Harry, your brother", or "This is a picture of Katy, your daughter, my, she was very little then!" or "My, don't we all change a lot over the years". This helps a person to "save face" if he/she can't recognise anyone, because we can just suggest that the people in the photos have changed a lot.
- When looking at a photo album with someone living with dementia, be particularly sensitive to the person's emotional response. Some people enjoy looking at photos of family and friends. For others, it produces unpleasant, nostalgic feelings which can be very upsetting.

- If the person shows any sign that he/she is not enjoying looking at the album or is getting upset by looking at the photos, bring the activity to a close and don't leave the person until you have restored emotional calm to him/her.
- Change the subject completely away from family and distract the person from unpleasant thoughts.
- Do not be put off by this experience. On another occasion, the person may enjoy looking at the very same album that they find upsetting today. Remember, all of us experience emotional highs and lows and people living with dementia are no different, in fact they are usually more prone to emotional highs and lows than the person who does not have dementia. So keep this in mind when showing family albums to a lady or gent with dementia.
- If the person has enjoyed looking at the album with you, thank the person and ask if he/she would like to look at it again some other day.

Motto
"Help me to remember where I come from."

GEOGRAPHY: (Where I Come From).

Aim: To help the person to "remember"
                                    where they come from and where they
                                    lived during their lifetime.

Activity: Flicking through an album of photos of
                                    the person's country, city or town as it
                                    evolved over the past 50 or 60 years.

Materials:
- A trolley on castors on which is placed:
- A scrapbook or album of photos, put together by someone who knows the person, i.e. a family member or friend.
- Labels under the photos with street names, city names or county names would be very useful.

Procedure:
- Approach the person in a friendly manner and greet him/her.
- Sit beside the person to his/her dominant side and introduce yourself.
- Ask, "May I show you this album?"
- If "yes", open it slowly at the first page and say, "I think this is an old picture of e.g. "Dublin City". (fill in the appropriate city).
- Allow the person to look at the picture.
- Then say, "Someone told me you come from Dublin". (fill in the correct city).
- Pointing to the picture say something like, "I think that's a picture of O'Connell Street".
- Pointing again to the picture say something like, "Are they trams in the street? my goodness, I'd forgotten they used to have trams in O'Connell Street".
- Allow the person time to recollect what "trams" were and how they themselves would have used them as transport in the past.
- Be ready to encourage any reminiscence that might be sparked off by looking at the picture. In this activity, conversation is a good thing, not a distraction.
- Pointing again to the picture say, "my goodness, look at those lamps, I think they're the old gas lamps they used to have in Dublin years ago."
- Again, allow the person plenty of time to recollect what gas lamps were and how they used to line the streets of Dublin (or other relevant city) years ago.

- Now, pointing to the picture again say, "And look at the horse drawn vans, I'd forgotten about those. Isn't it amazing how things have changed," you'd never see a horse drawn van now".
- Once you've started the flow of conversation, allow the person to start joining in.
- Be observant of the person's demeanour. Try to make sure the activity is producing a positive and not a negative effect.
- If the person is becoming too nostalgic or even tearful, carefully bring the activity to a close.
- Change the subject matter. Do not leave the person until his/her emotional state has been stabilised.
- Do not be disheartened. Nostalgia is a fact of life. On another occasion, the person may enjoy flicking through this book of old photos.
- If the person is enjoying the activity, continue on until you come to the end of the album or scrapbook and feel free to engage the person in any conversation that gets sparked off from looking at the photos.
- Finally, thank the person for his/her co-operation and ask if he/she would like to look through the album on another day.
- Finish by putting away the album and maybe inviting the person to have a cup of tea with you.
- If conversation continues, be ready to encourage it and make sure the activity ends on a positive note.

Motto
"Help me to remember the hobbies I enjoyed."

HOBBIES:	(What I loved to do).
Activity:	D.I.Y.
Preliminary Activity:	Hammering wooden pegs into a wooden pegboard.
Aim:	To "jog" the person's "muscular memory" so as to re-activate the person's "subconscious ability" to use a hammer.
Motto:	"Prime the pump."

Materials:
- A trolley on castors on which is placed:
- A tray containing:
- A wooden pegboard.
- A box containing 20 wooden pegs.
- A wooden hammer.

Procedure:
- Approach the person in a friendly manner and greet him.
- Sit beside the person to his dominant side and introduce yourself.
- Ask, "Can I show you this activity?"
- Take the tray and place it either on a table or on the person's lap.
- Slowly and deliberately, pick up a wooden peg.
- Slowly and deliberately, lift up the hammer.
- Slowly and carefully, hold the peg over one of the holes in the pegboard and begin to hammer the peg into the hole.
- Repeat.
- Now, indicate to the person that it is his turn to hammer in a peg.
- Hand the hammer to the person.
- Allow him sufficient time to work out what he has to do.
- When he has hammered in one peg, gesture to him to hammer in some more.
- When all the pegs are hammered in say something like, "Well done, great job".
- Finally, thank the person and ask if he enjoyed the activity.
- Inquire whether he would like to do the activity again, on another occasion.

Motto
"Encourage me to resume the hobbies I enjoyed."

HOBBIES:	(What I loved to do).
Activity:	D.I.Y.
Target Activity:	Hammering real nails into wood to fix things, such as garden fencing or household furniture.
Aim:	To re-activate and fix into a habit, the person's procedural ability to use a hammer.
Goal:	To motivate the person to engage in meaningful activity, i.e. "work" and to take an interest in caring for his own environment by doing light handyman activities.

Materials:
- A tray on which is placed:
- A wooden hammer (lightweight).
- A box with 4 nails. (not too small as that might present a choking hazard).
- A wooden stool that has an x marked in pencil at the 4 points that need a nail hammered in and that has pre-drilled holes to make hammering easier.
-

Procedure:
- Approach the person in a friendly manner and greet him.
- Sit beside him to his dominant side and introduce yourself.
- Ask, "Could you help me to fix this stool?"
- If "yes", slowly reach for a nail out of the box.
- Next, slowly and deliberately, reach for the hammer.
- Slowly and deliberately, hold the nail over the stool at the point marked x and, lifting the hammer, start to hammer in the nail.
- Try not to talk as this will take the focus off the activity. Hammer the nail in.
- Now, indicate that it is the person's turn to hammer a nail in.
- Observe carefully, as the person places the nail into position.
- Observe vigilantly, as the person hammers in the nail, making sure he does not do anything to hurt himself.
- When all 4 nails have been hammered in, say, "great job, you've fixed the stool".

Montessori for Dementia.

Motto
"Help me to remember the hobbies I enjoyed."

HOBBIES:	(What I loved to do).
Activity:	Sewing
Preliminary Activity:	Using metal tipped laces and sewing cards.
Aim:	To "jog" the person's "muscular memory" so as to re-activate the person's "subconscious ability" to use a needle and thread.
Motto:	"Prime the Pump".
Goal:	To motivate the person to to engage in meaningful activity, i.e. "work".

Materials:
- A tray.
- 2 sewing cards.
- 2 metal tipped laces.

Procedure:
- Approach the person in a friendly manner, greet her and introduce yourself.
- Ask, "could you help me with these sewing cards?"
- If "yes", take a metal tipped lace and slowly and deliberately push the metal point into a hole in the sewing card.
- Pull the lace all the way through the hole.
- Now, pass a sewing card and a lace to the lady.
- Say, "Would you like to sew this one?"
- If the lady seems confused about what to do, teach by doing, not by talking, i.e take your own metal tipped lace and slowly and deliberately push the metal tip into a hole in the sewing card, then pull the lace all the way through the hole, as before.
- Always make sure your movements are slow and deliberate and easy to follow.
- Remember not to talk too much, because talk will distract the person, causing her to loose focus.
- When the card has been "sewed", thank the person for her co-operation.
- Ask if she would like to do the activity again, sometime.

Motto
"Encourage me to resume the hobbies I enjoyed."

HOBBIES:	(What I loved to do).
Activity:	Sewing
Target Activity:	Using a needle and thread..
Aim:	To reactivate and fix into a routine the person's "procedural ability" to perform the physical actions involved in their former hobby of sewing.
Goal:	To motivate the person to engage in meaningful activity, i.e. "work".

Materials:
- A tray.
- A sewing kit containing :
- 2 blunt-ended plastic sewing needles, already threaded with bright thread.
- 2 sewing/embroidery squares with a simple drawing etched on them, i.e a sunflower.
-

Procedure:
- Approach the person in a friendly manner and greet her.
- Sit beside the person and introduce yourself.
- Ask, "Could you help me to do some sewing?"
- If "yes", take one of the sewing sheets in your left hand, and take a blunt-ended plastic needle and thread in your right hand, and slowly and deliberately, push the needle through one of the holes in the sewing sheet.
- Now pull the needle and thread all the way through the hole.
- Next, pass the other sewing/embroidery sheet to the person.
- Say, "Could you sew this one please?"
- If the person seems confused, once again, teach by doing, not talking, i.e take your own needle and thread and slowly and deliberately, almost in slow motion, push the needle into a hole in the sewing/embroidery sheet.
- Always make sure your movements are slow and deliberate and easy to follow.
- Remember to keep all talking to a minimum as "talk" may confuse or distract the person, causing him/her to lose focus.
- When the sewing is finished, thank the person and ask if he/she would like to do more sewing another day.

Montessori for Dementia.

Motto
"Help me to remember the music I loved."

MUSIC :   (What I liked to listen to).

Aim: To help the person to "remember" the music he/she used to enjoy.

Activities: 1. Playing a musical instrument.
                                         2. Listening to music on a C.D.

Materials:
- 1) A musical instrument similar to the instrument the person used to play.
- 2) A compact disc player and some C.D.s of music you think the person would be familiar with from the past.

Procedure for Activity 1.
- Approach the person in a friendly manner and greet him/her.
- Sit beside the person to their dominant side and introduce yourself.
- Ask, "Would you like to see this keyboard player I have brought with me?"
- Bring the person (who may be in a wheel-chair) over to the keyboard.
- Switch the keyboard on and play a simple tune.
- Say, "I hear you used to play the piano, would you like to have a go at this?"
- If "yes", place the keyboard in front of you and the person on a table or stand.
- Switch on the keyboard and play a pre-programmed tune. Say, "sounds good".
- Give the person time to acclimatise then invite him/her to start playing.
- When the person starts playing, be careful not to talk or do anything to take his/her focus off playing the keyboard.
- Encourage him/her to play a few pieces.
- When he/she is finished say, "wow, that was really great."
- Ask the person if he/she enjoyed playing the instrument. If the person is chatty, ask about what other instruments he/she may have played in the past.
- Finally, thank the person and ask if you could do this again sometime.

Procedure for Activity 2.
- Follow the first and second steps in the procedure above .
- Ask, "Would you like to listen to some music/songs with me?"
- If "yes", turn on the compact disc player and start playing the music/songs.
- Observe the person's response. If he/she is enjoying the music keep playing it.
- Clap or sing along if appropriate. If the person starts to chat be responsive.
- Thank the person and inquire if he/she would like to do this again sometime.

Cultural Activities

Motto
"Help me to remember what kept me active."

MOVEMENT: (What kept me active).

Aim: To help the person to "remember" the physical activities they used to enjoy.

Activities: Examples:
1) Swaying, tapping , dancing to music.
2) Cleaning golf clubs.
3) Sorting fishing tackle.
4) Cleaning bicycle lamps, bell, etc.
5) Cleaning hiking boots,walking shoes.

Materials: (for example 4)
- 1 box containing:
- 2 bicycle lamps that need cleaning.
- 2 bicycle bells that need cleaning.
- 2 cleaning cloths.

Procedure:
- Approach the person in a friendly manner and sit beside him/her.
- Greet the person and introduce yourself.
- Say, "I hear you used to cycle a lot when you were younger."
- Ask, "Could I show you what I've got here?"
- If "yes", open the box and take out the two bicycle lamps.
- Say, "These are two bicycle lamps. They are very dusty, could you clean one for me and I'll clean the other?"
- If "yes", pass a duster to the person, and keep one for yourself.
- Pass a lamp to the person.
- Take the other lamp yourself and slowly and deliberately start dusting it.
- Indicate to the person to do the same.
- Initially, avoid talking as this could confuse the person, but if the activity sparks memories in the person, relating to their cycling days (or anything else), be prepared to encourage this kind of conversation.
- When the lamps are cleaned ask the person to help you to clean the bells.
- When everything has been cleaned, thank the person for his/her help.
- Ask the person if he/she would like to do this again some other time.

Montessori for Dementia.

Motto
"Help me to celebrate my heritage."

HERITAGE: (What I identified With).

Aim: To help the person to "remember" his/
                                                  her heritage.

Activity: Flicking through a tailor-made
                                                  scrapbook containing memorabilia
                                                  relating to the person's heritage.

Materials:
- A trolley on castors on which is placed:
- A cardboard box containing:
- 2 x St. Patrick's Day cards.
- 2 x St. Patrick's Day badges with tricolour ribbons on them.
- 2 x small Irish flags.
- 2 x pictures of a St. Patrick's Day parade.
- 2 x pictures of leprechauns.
- 1 x CD of traditional Irish music.
- 1 x CD player.

Procedure:
- Approach the person in a friendly manner and greet him/her.
- Sit beside the person to his/her dominant side and introduce yourself.
- Ask, "Would you like to see what I've got here?"
- If "yes" open the cardboard box and take out a St. Patrick's Day card, (preferably one with a large green shamrock on it rather than small pictures).
- Say something like, "This is a St. Patrick's Day card".
- Allow the person plenty of time to examine the card.
- Next take out an Irish flag and , holding it by the wooden pole, wave it a little.
- Now, pass it to the person for him/her to wave.
- Say, "I think people wave these at the St. Patrick's Day parade".
- Allow the person time to register what you are saying. He/she may feel prompted to reply or even to recollect waving flags themselves at a parade.
- Next, take out a St. Patrick's Day badge with a tricolour ribbon on it.
- Pin it on your chest and proudly show the person its purpose.

- Take out the other badge and invite the person to pin it on him/her.
- Take out another flag and together with the person wave the flags while wearing the badges.
- If the person appears to be enjoying the game ask, "would you like to hear some Irish music?"
- If "yes", put the CD into the player and play a song.
- Wave the flags while the music plays.
- Now, take out some of the photos of St. Patrick's Day parades and show them to the person.
- When the the song is finished, ask the person if he/she would like to hear some more songs.
- If "yes," continue but be careful not to exhaust the person.
- If "no", pack up quietly, thank the person and say something like, "it was really lovely spending time with you, maybe we could do this again another time".

Montessori for Dementia.

HISTORY: (What I Lived Through).

Aim: To help the person to "remember" his/her place in time.

Activity: Flicking through a tailor-made scrap book containing memorabilia relating to important historical events which occurred during the person's lifetime.

Materials:
- A trolley on which is placed:
- A scrapbook containing newspaper cuttings from the 1930s to the present day. These could be copies of newspaper headlines relating to historical events which would have had real significance for this particular person. This scrapbook needs to be put together by people who knew or still know the person well. For example, a scrapbook with newspaper clippings relating to World War 1 and "Poppy Day" will have great significance for a British elderly person who may have lost relatives in this Great War but will probably have less significance for a person from a country which had less direct involvement in the war. The scrapbook could contain some clippings of events which evoked worldwide interest such as the assassinations of President J.F. Kennedy and Dr. Martin Luther King. Happier events, such as the coronation of Queen Elizabeth 11 and years later the wedding of Lady Diana to Prince Charles could also be recorded.

Procedure:
- Approach the person in a friendly manner and greet him/her.
- Sit beside the person to his/her dominant side and introduce yourself.
- Ask, "May I show you this scrapbook I put together ?"
- If "yes", open the book at page 1 and comment on the newspaper cuttings.
- Try to get conversation flowing, but remember to give the person plenty of time to get their thoughts together and put them into speech.
- Be observant about what photos or newspaper clippings arouse the most interest in the person.
- Continue through the scrapbook if the person shows an interest.
- Finally, thank the person and ask if you could do this again sometime.

Motto
"Help me to celebrate my traditions."

TRADITIONS: (What I Celebrate)

Aim: To help the person to "remember" the traditions that played an important part in their lives.

Activities: Examples.
1) Christmas Activities.
2) Easter Activities.
3) Thanksgiving.
4) Forth of July Celebrations.
5) Jewish Festivals.
6) Hindu Festivals.
7) Islamic Festivals.

Materials:
(For Christmas Activities).
- A trolley on castors containing:
- A tray with xmas tree decorations which all have large, easily visible ,hooks.
- The decorations should be laid out on the tray in an orderly fashion.
-

Procedure:
- Approach the person in a friendly manner and greet him/her.
- Sit beside the person and introduce yourself.
- Ask. "Could you help me to decorate the Christmas tree?"
- If "yes", take the person, who may be in a wheelchair over to the Christmas tree.
- Say, "We need to put these decorations on the tree".
- Take a Christmas tree decoration and slowly and deliberately, hang it on the Christmas tree.
- Say, "Wow, that looks lovely".
- Now, hand a Christmas tree decoration to the person.
- Say, "Could you hang your decoration on this branch". (pointing to a branch).
- Allow the person plenty of time to register what you are indicating.
- When the person has done this, take another decoration and repeat as above.
- When all the decorations have been placed on the tree, say, "We've done well!"
- Ask the person if he/she enjoyed the activity.
- Now invite the person to have a cup of tea with you and a few xmas cookies, (cut into Christmas tree shapes, if possible).

Montessori for Dementia.

Motto
"Help me to remember what I believe."

SPIRITUALITY: (What gave me hope and meaning)

Aim: To "subliminally" aid the person to remember the spirituality they once engaged in.

Activities: (Indirect Approach:)

In the person's hearing,

Preliminary Activities:
1) Play hymns in the background.
2) Put religious services on television.
3) Read religious books out loud.

Materials:
- C.D.s of religious music. These could be traditional hymns which would be ingrained in the memory of any person who was a church-goer in the 1930s, 1940s, 1950s, 1960s or 1970s. After this time, hymns changed substantially.
- A television which transmits religious programmes from around the world.
- A person willing to sit near the person and read from religious books.

Procedure:
(For a family member caring for a person with dementia, in his/her own home).
- Find out what hymns would have been most familiar to the person with dementia when they were younger.
- Get a C.D. of those hymns.
- When the person is resting or even sleeping, play the C.D. in the background.
- Later, say to the person, "I was playing some hymns earlier, did you like them?"
- If "yes", ask could you play some more.
-

Procedure:
(For care staff caring for a person living with dementia in a care facility).
- Follow the first and second steps as above.
- When the person is in his/her own room, (not the common sitting room), play the C.D. of hymns as background music.
- Another time, play a religious programme on a T.V. in the person's room.
- On another occasion, play a tape or get someone to read the scriptures to the person either while he/she is resting in a chair or even while he/she is sleeping. The spirit never sleeps, so a person can absorb spiritual food even when asleep.
- When the person is awake, say, "I read some scripture to you while you were resting, would you like me to do that again, another day?" If "yes", do that.

Motto
"Allow me to celebrate what I believe."

SPIRITUALITY: (What gave me hope and meaning)

Goal: To motivate the person to participate in spiritual life once more.

Activities: (Direct Approach)

Target Activity: 1) Attending religious services.
2) Singing hymns.
3) Praying in services and at home.
4) Reading scripture.
5) Attending church social events.

Materials:
- A kind individual willing to transport the person to religious services. Or,
- A pastor /priest willing to bring the religious services to the person.
- Individuals willing to arrange dementia friendly, informal sessions in the person's home/care home, where hymns will be sung, prayers will be said and scriptures will be read aloud.
- Individuals willing to arrange dementia friendly, church social events where persons living with dementia can continue to be part of the church family.

Procedure:
(For care staff caring for a person living with dementia in a care facility).
- Arrange for 3 or 4 church-goers to come to the care home to conduct an informal religious service.
- Prepare a room in the care home which is quite and church like. Arrange suitable seating for the persons with dementia and make sure there is a toilet nearby and a care worker to help with toileting, if necessary.
- Keep the format simple. A good start would be to have someone announce slowly and clearly that this is a church service, we will sing one hymn, read from the Bible and say a prayer. Then we will finish with tea and cake.
- The words of the hymn should be written in large print and clearly displayed.
- The passage from the Bible should be in large print and clearly displayed.
- When the service is finished, the remaining skills of the residents should be utilised to the full. A person able to pour soft drinks, should be invited to do that. A person able to pass around a plate of cup cakes, should be invited to do that. A person able to fold napkins and/or pass them out should be invited to do that. A person able to collect cups on a trolley, should be invited to do that.
- All persons should be thanked for coming and invited to come again.

EXTENSIONS TO THE CULTURAL ACTIVITIES:

To preserve the person's connection to the things that made up his/her cultural life, encourage activities with the following Montessori inspired materials:

FAMILY: Family Tree classification cards.

GEOGRAPHY: "Where I come from" classification cards.

HOBBIES: "The things I loved to do" classification cards.

MUSIC: "The music I loved" classification cards.

MOVEMENT: "The activities I enjoyed" classification cards.

HERITAGE: "My heritage" classification cards.

HISTORY: "The events I lived through" classification cards.

TRADITIONS: "The traditions I loved" classification cards.

SPIRITUALITY: "The hymns I loved" classification cards.

D.I.Y. Hint.

The cards should be made in conjunction with a family member or friend of the person, who is very familiar with the person's background, likes, dislikes etc.

The cards could be made from photographs or pictures cut from magazines. They should be laminated and/or glued onto hard card. There should be an A4 control card for each category. Each category should be kept in a separate box.

CONCLUSION

"Nothing can take the place of work.......work is an inherent tendency
in human nature, it is the characteristic instinct of the human race."

(The Secret of Childhood p200)
Dr. Maria Montessori.

In her long life, Dr. Maria Montessori discovered many important facts about the human condition. Perhaps the most important fact she discovered was the necessity for "work", i.e. meaningful activity, for the mental health and well-being of all humans.

Dr. Montessori recognised that young children, adolescents, and even adults display all sorts of negative behaviours, some mild, some severe, but she was convinced that they all come under one heading and that is "deviations". She was certain that the myriad of negative behaviours seen in human beings are simply "deviations" from the normal course of development.

Furthermore, she was certain that all deviations have one common source. They all result from "obstacles" which stand in the way of a person's capacity to follow the laws of life, one of which is the "law of work".

When the human being is deprived of his/her natural urge to "work", i.e. to carry out meaningful activity, something very sinister occurs in his/her personality, i.e he/she "deviates" from normality and a myriad of negative personality traits emerge.

This, we believe is exactly what happens when people develop dementia. When a person no longer has opportunities to carry out meaningful activity, slowly but surely, negative behaviours, often called "responsive behaviours" begin to appear.

It is interesting that just as Dr. Montessori identified different types of deviation in children depending upon their personality dispositions, (strong/week), so too can we identify different types of deviation or "responsive behaviours" in persons living with dementia, depending on their personality type.

People who have a strong or "dominant" personality type often display aggressive behaviour. They scream, shout, bang and hit. People who have a weak or "submissive" personality type often show sadness, apathy, depression and reluctance to take part in anything. Although, much of this behaviour is caused by the medical condition that is dementia, it is nonetheless a sign of "deviation" and the source of it is always the same. It is caused by obstacles which prevent the person from engaging in meaningful activity, i.e "work".

So, what's the cure? Well, Dr. Montessori found that, in young children, all deviations could be cured by a phenomenon she came to call "normalisation through work". She eventually said the discovery of "normalisation through work" was

> "the most important single result of our whole work".
>
> (The Absorbent Mind p204)
>
> Dr. Maria Montessori.

We believe that a type of normalisation, (unfortunately, not as dramatic as that seen in the child under six years), is possible in people living with dementia, and that this "normalisation", once again, comes about through meaningful activity, i.e "work".

So, instead of focusing on "responsive behaviours" and trying to come up with solutions to cope with them, we believe the correct approach is to ignore the "responsive behaviours" and focus on meaningful activity i.e "work" and how we can motivate people living with dementia to engage in it.

If we can do this, we will see many of the "responsive behaviours" just disappearing and being replaced by positive behaviours such as engagement in activity, focus and concentration, persistence and application to a task.

These positive behaviours, in turn, lead to success in the carrying out of tasks and success in itself leads to an increase in self-esteem.

All of this creates a cycle of positivity because increased self-esteem leads to a happier human being and a happier human being has a better quality of life. But it doesn't stop there. A better quality of life for the person living with dementia has a positive knock on effect, not just for the person living with dementia, but also for their caregivers, family and friends and it ultimately gives them too, a better quality of life.

It is for this reason, that Montessori-Based Activity for people living with dementia is now being described as a "game-changer" in the world of dementia care.

ABOUT THE AUTHORS

"Once these facts have been seen, one cannot cease from writing and talking about them."   Dr. Maria Montessori.

Stephen and Bernadette Phillips have been involved in Montessori education and research for over 30 years. They have enjoyed practicing, lecturing and writing about all things Montessori for most of their adult lives.

Stephen is originally from Wiltshire, in England and Bernadette is from Dublin, Ireland.

In recent years they have been very much focused on the pioneering research of Dr. Cameron Camp into Montessori-Based Programmes for people living with dementia.

Having run Montessori schools for years, they now work as independent Montessori consultants.

They give workshops on Montessori principles and practice, covering infancy, childhood, adolescence and early adulthood.

They also give seminars and workshops on Montessori-Based Programmes for people living with dementia.

They can be contacted at the following e-mail addresses:

bernadette_phillips@yahoo.co.uk

sendsteveane@yahoo.co.uk

Made in the USA
Las Vegas, NV
24 September 2021